Primary Care
of the Elderly:
A Practical Approach

J. WILLIAMSON CBE, MB ChB, FRCPE
Head of the Department of Geriatric Medicine, University of Edinburgh
Professor Emeritus, Geriatric Medicine, University of Edinburgh

R. G. SMITH MB ChB FRCPE
Senior Lecturer in Geriatric Medicine, University of Edinburgh

L. E. BURLEY MB ChB FRCPE MRCGP
Consultant Physician in Geriatric Medicine, East Fortune Hospital,
East Lothian

With a Foreword by
A. G. DONALD OBE, FRCPE, FRCGP
Formerly Chairman, Royal College of General Practitioners; Regional
Adviser in General Practice, South-East Scotland; Assistant Director,
Edinburgh Postgraduate Board

WRIGHT
Bristol
1987

Published under the Wright imprint by
IOP Publishing Limited
Techno House, Redcliffe Way, Bristol BS1 6NX

British Library Cataloguing in Publication Data
Williamson, J.
    Primary care of the elderly: a practical
    approach.
    1. Geriatrics 2. Family medicine
    I. Title II. Smith, R. G. (Roger G.)
    III. Burley, Lindsay
    618.97   RC952

ISBN 0 7236 0633 1

Typeset by
BC Typesetting
51 School Road, Oldland Common, Bristol BS15 6PJ

Printed in Great Britain by
The Bath Press, Lower Bristol Road, Bath BA2 3BL.

(19.95

FIE

PR_____ ___ ___ HE ELDERLY:
A PRACTICAL APPROACH

Preface

In the past few years the University Department of Geriatric Medicine has collaborated with the Edinburgh Postgraduate Board for Medicine in running courses for primary health care providers. Our objectives were numerous but we identified two major requirements:

1. To define the topics which form the major problems for general practitioners, and
2. To determine the best forms of learning in these areas.

We were in no doubt at the outset that Professor Bernard Isaacs' *Giants of Geriatrics** had already covered a very large part of the field. These are mental confusion, falls, reduced mobility and incontinence, and they have provided the main basis for our courses. However, we soon realized that two other clinical topics had to be included: strokes and drugs and prescribing problems. We also found it useful to include a session on the special needs of the aged patient and how to identify them and so Chapter 1 deals with this general topic. We have also covered Case Finding in General Practice and since the topic has come up repeatedly in the courses, we conclude with a chapter on Services for the Elderly, especially how the primary care team should relate to them.

In our courses we have used case histories and illustrative clinical and family situations as much as possible in the expectation that this would stimulate discussion and argument.

Another decision which we took at the outset was that we would not invite 'subspecialists' to contribute to these courses. Instead the three of us presented our material to the group reinforced, where possible, by others directly involved with elderly patients, e.g. general practitioner colleagues, relatives, nurses, rehabilitation therapists and social workers. It was hoped that participants would benefit from hearing the views of these other groups more than they would from hearing from more highly specialized medically qualified persons. We believe that this objective was often achieved and each of us certainly learned much from hearing and seeing these individuals, all of whom are closely involved with older persons. We have tried to incorporate this experience here.

* Bernard Isaacs, *Giants of Geriatrics: A Study of Symptoms in Old Age.* University of Birmingham, 1976.

Arising from this experience, we felt that it would be useful to produce a small book which, in dealing with these topics in this way, would be of help to trainee general practitioners (and their senior colleagues) by giving them a better appreciation of the problems of their elderly patients and the difficulties experienced by their families in attempting to support them. We also hope that it will be of help not only to other professionals in the primary care team, but also to all those whose work brings them into contact with elderly patients.

J. W.
R. G. S.
L. E. B.

Contents

Foreword

The impact of an ageing population has borne particularly heavily on primary care. Not only the general practitioner, but the nurse, the health visitor, the social worker and the home help shoulder greater responsibilities in their efforts to meet the essential requirements of a service for the care of the elderly. That requirement is to provide, with the help of our specialist colleagues, an integrated and skilled service to support the elderly in independence, comfort and contentment in their own homes, for as long as possible.

During the past twenty years it has been a pleasure for me as a general practitioner to observe the development of such an integrated service, and the Scottish achievement in this field is one of which we can be justifiably proud. I have been privileged to observe, and to work with, Professor James Williamson and his colleagues over these years and they have taught me a great deal. They have earned the gratitude not only of general practitioners, but most importantly of patients, by the caring and skilled service which they have been instrumental in developing—demonstrating as it has holistic care at its best.

Therefore it gives me great pleasure to commend this book to all who are charged with any aspect of caring for the elderly in primary care.

ALASTAIR G. DONALD
OBE, FRCPE, FRCGP

1 THE NATURE OF NEED IN OLD AGE

Effective health care of old patients involves the detection of their needs and then meeting these needs by provision of services and resources as speedily and economically as possible. In old age it is essential to include family members and other supporters since in a large majority it is the family unit which we have to protect and strengthen. Hence the needs of family members must also be identified and met. This is often a very complex matter and identified needs may vary from simple social support for a lonely old person to the provision of several community services, plus detailed clinical diagnosis involving the full panoply of modern medical technology.

Medicine of old age thus is not just 'whole person medicine' but is indeed family medicine in its most real form. Support for relatives is an essential part of good care since if they are over-extended or taken beyond their limits of tolerance, all experience shows that their willingness and ability to continue a supporting role may collapse and rejection will occur. This is, unfortunately, often an irreversible breakdown.

ASSESSMENT OF NEED AND DIAGNOSIS

Traditionally, medical diagnosis has meant that the lesion was localized and its pathological nature determined. This process, of course, applies in old age but is often more complex because older patients tend to have multiple diseases both physical and mental.

Hence the medical diagnosis has to be very thorough with careful history taking and systematic examination. In addition to this medical diagnosis we have to include in our assessment the patient's functional capacity and sources of support and help. It will be clear to the reader that once we stray outside the limits of traditional clinico-pathological diagnosis then we may very soon need the help and expertise of other professions, especially nurses, therapists and social workers. Effective health care of the old therefore frequently necessitates teamwork and

1

general practitioners should be encouraged to see themselves as team members. This means the achievement of good working relations and effective communication with colleagues in the above disciplines. A good geriatric service is, of course, essential in providing optimum care for the elderly and support for their families and also to ensure the most effective and economical use of resources, which will always be in short supply because of the continuous process of ageing of the population. General practitioners and their community nursing colleagues should therefore be encouraged to visit their local department of geriatric medicine and to get to know the staff there.

DEMOGRAPHIC TRENDS

The ageing of populations which has occurred this century is well known and we shall only comment here upon the more important trends.

1. The steep increase in the number of persons aged 65 and above is now nearly over and from 1990 this group will remain fairly constant into the twenty-first century.
2. The rapid increase which has occurred in the 75+ group will continue till the end of this century and thereafter remain fairly constant.
3. The 85+ group will continue to increase right up to the year 2021 (which is as far as the Registrar General has forecast).
4. The ratio of females to males in the population increases with age. For the group aged 85+ it is about 5:2.

Although it is unsatisfactory to use age alone as a predictor of need, the implications of these demographic data are most important for general practitioners since they will be increasingly involved with aged patients, especially females.

The demands upon primary care from elderly patients are disproportionately high because of the increased levels of sickness and dependency in this age group. *Table* 1.1 shows the approximate numbers of patients in a UK practice of 2500 patients in each age group.

The amount of work associated with different age groups is shown in *Fig.* 1.1 with patients aged 70 and over having the highest consultation rates.

It is most proper that the great bulk of medical care of older patients should continue to be provided by general practitioners, and for those who are well versed in such care and working in a smoothly functioning primary care team there is great satisfaction to be had in meeting this challenge. Conversely, general practitioners who are not suitably prepared (in terms of knowledge, skills and attitudes) will experience poor professional satisfaction and frustration as demands increase and performance falters.

Table 1.1. No. of patients by age in a practice of 2500

Age group	No. of persons
0–14	620
15–44	1000
45–64	500
65–74	250
75 +	130

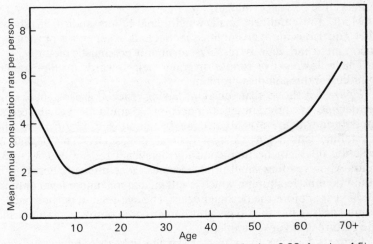

Mean annual consultation rates by age group (males: 3·33; females: 4·5)

Fig. 1.1. Mean annual consultation rates by age group. (*Reproduced* by kind permission of Dr John Fry and MTP Press Ltd.)

This book has been produced with the aim of helping practitioners to understand the nature of need in old age, how to identify it and how to meet it.

FUNCTION IN RELATION TO AGE

The usual representation of how function changes with age is shown in *Fig.* 1.2 which portrays three phases of development.

1. *Growth*, starting at birth with very low levels of function and low functional reserves. Rapid increase follows as biological vigour increases.
2. *Maturity*, when growth has ceased and function is at its maximum. At this stage there are large reserves of function and the individual can withstand severe stress such as physical exertion, injury and intercurrent illness. This phase is traditionally portrayed as a brief plateau preceding descent into the next phase.
3. *Senescence*, in which there is a linear decline in function and functional reserves are progressively reduced.

From *Fig*. 1.2 it will be seen that, from birth onwards, there is increasing variability. This explains the common observation that some individuals at 70 appear fitter and have superior function to others 20 or 25 years younger.

Modern research, especially longitudinal cohort studies, has shown that *Fig*. 1.2 is an oversimplified model and in general it presents an incomplete and, in most respects, an unduly pessimistic picture.

The following five simple diagrams help towards a fuller understanding of this complex problem.

Figure 1.3 shows that function, having reached a peak, may start to decline at different ages. Function A could be visual accommodation which starts to decline by about age 12 or 13 as the crystalline lens begins to show decreased elasticity. This decline in function does not become clinically significant for another 30 or 35 years when reading small print becomes more difficult. Function B could be muscle strength which is retained at maximum level until 25 or 30 years before the decline begins. The age-related decline once it commences is linear in type. But humans are complex creatures and the picture is never so simple.

Figure 1.4 shows the effect of starting unhealthy behaviour, e.g. cigarette smoking at, say, age 18. This will lead to increased loss of respiratory and cardiac function so that the curve will be steeper than in *Fig*. 1.3. On the contrary, the adoption of healthier behaviour may improve function. This has been recently shown to be possible even in old age, and a Swedish controlled experiment with 70-year-old men showed that simple physical exercise was associated with marked improvement in function and fitness (as shown by increased maximum oxygen consumption and muscle strength and reduction in the increase in heart rate after submaximal exercise).

Environmental influences during the lifespan will also affect function. Thus the individual who has been reared in an industrially polluted environment will suffer and respiratory and other functions might be impaired as a result.

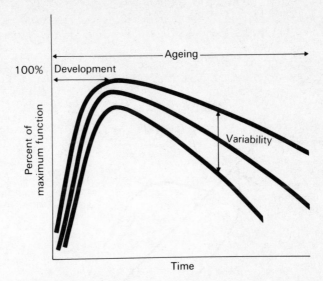

Fig. 1.2. Function in relation to age.

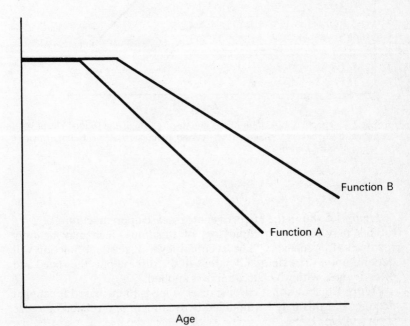

Fig. 1.3. Function in relation to age. (*Reproduced* by kind permission of the Editor, *Nova Scotia Medical Bulletin*.)

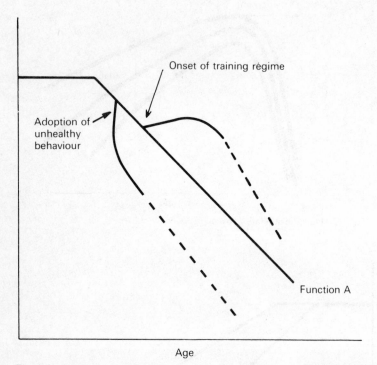

Fig. 1.4. Function in relation to age and disease. Modifying factors: Healthy/ unhealthy behaviour. (*Reproduced* by kind permission of the Editor, *Nova Scotia Medical Bulletin*.)

Figure 1.5 shows the effect of acute disease upon function.

This may lead to a rapid loss of function which may be fully restored after recovery. The eventual level of residual function will depend upon the extent and nature of the disease plus the speed and effectiveness with which treatment is applied.

Figure 1.6 shows that chronic disease leads to increased functional decline, but this may be modified by treatment and rehabilitation as shown in *Fig*. 1.7.

These five diagrams indicate clearly that the picture is almost infinitely varied from individual to individual and the functional status

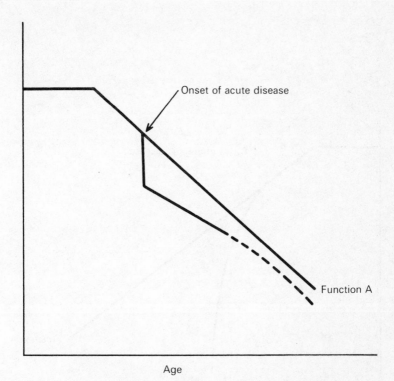

Fig. 1.5. Function in relation to age. Modifying factors: Effects of acute disease.
(*Reproduced* by kind permission of the Editor, *Nova Scotia Medical Bulletin.*)

of any elderly person is determined by the interplay of four chief factors. These are (1) heredity, (2) changes due to age alone, (3) changes due to disease, and (4) changes associated with behavioural and environmental factors.

The thoughtful reader may have noticed that medicine has tended to be concerned mainly (sometimes exclusively) with item (3), i.e. pathological diagnosis. We would like to emphasize that such a limited approach is inadequate in old age and often will give an incomplete assessment of patients' needs.

We shall now consider each of these factors in turn.

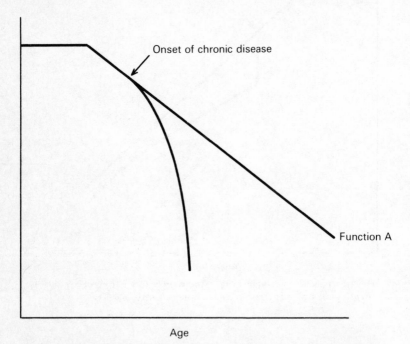

Fig. 1.6. Function in relation to age. Modifying factors: Chronic disease. (*Reproduced* by kind permission of the Editor, *Nova Scotia Medical Bulletin.*)

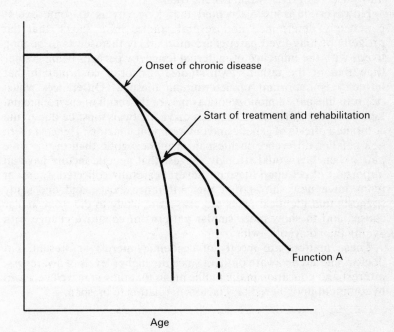

Fig. 1.7. Function in relation to age. Modifying factors: Chronic disease, treatment and rehabilitation. (*Reproduced* by kind permission of the Editor, *Nova Scotia Medical Bulletin.*)

HEREDITY

It is a matter of common observation that individuals belonging to certain families age more slowly than others. There are so many factors involved and measurement of biological age (as opposed to chronological age) is so imprecise that scientific proof of this observation is lacking. Thus members of the same family are likely to have experienced similar favourable or unfavourable behavioural or environmental influences such as diet, exposure to communicable disease or exposure to atmospheric pollution, and these influences may obscure or overwhelm genetic traits.

However, it is now accepted that longevity is to some extent genetically determined and several studies have shown that the progeny of long-lived parents are more likely themselves to be long lived, with the influence of maternal longevity perhaps being greater than that of the father. Twin studies also offer confirmation that heredity is important in determining lifespan. Differences which occur in lifespan of monozygotic twins are the result of environmental factors, while differences between dizygotic twins must be due to the combined effects of genetic and environmental factors. Hence if there is a smaller difference in lifespan in monozygotic than in dizygotic pairs, then this would strongly suggest that genetic factors have an important effect upon lifespan. Several carefully collected studies of twins have now shown that this difference exists, and one study suggests that identical twins are also more likely to die from similar causes and to show more similar patterns of cognitive change with ageing than dizygotic twins.

These matters are mostly of academic interest at present, but doctors should be aware of them since the higher levels of awareness, interest and education in the public mean that they may well be asked to comment upon hereditary factors in relation to lifespan.

AGE CHANGES

All living organisms show changes due to the ageing process and these occur at molecular, cellular, organ and organismal levels. Much research effort has been expended in trying to elucidate the mechanisms involved in the production of age changes. So far, however, no single theory has proved acceptable and the current view is that several factors are involved in the ageing process.

Although we are largely ignorant of the causes and mechanisms of ageing, we do know a great deal about its effects. As already explained, each function appears to reach its zenith at a certain age, is maintained for a time and then undergoes decline in a linear fashion.

We are, however, so generously endowed with surplus function that we are generally unaware of this functional age-related decline until we are well beyond middle age. Functional reserves are, nevertheless, steadily eroded with the passage of time and for the increasing numbers who survive into extreme old age (75+ to 85+), then age changes *per se* may lead to significant reductions in functional reserves. Thus, if as seems to be the case, renal function declines by at least 1 per cent per year from age 25 onwards, by age 85 we may have lost 60 per cent or more of our renal function *by age changes alone*. If prostatism, recurrent urinary tract infection or nephrosclerosis have taken their toll as well, then the renal reserves in an 85-year-old patient may be very meagre or close to zero.

It is inappropriate here to attempt to detail age changes in different systems; some will be mentioned in ensuing chapters as they relate to the topics being discussed.

Modern research, especially that based upon longitudinal studies, has tended to show that, in disease-free subjects, the plateau of function at the phase of maturity is much more prolonged than previously believed (and as portrayed in *Fig.* 1.2). This good news applies equally to physical and mental functions.

DISEASE CHANGES

Figures 1.4 and 1.5 above show how function may decline suddenly with acute or chronic disease, and if this occurs in an individual in whom significant functional decline due to age already exists then organ reserves may rapidly approach zero. Hence any stress may produce organ failure, and if one organ fails due to stress the extra load thrust upon other compromised organs may lead to a knock-on effect and multiple system failure.

Atypical Presentation of Disease

The clinical medicine of old age is made more complex by the fact that disease in old age often presents in an atypical fashion, and the description of disease presentation in medical textbooks may not apply. The manifestations of acute disease tend to be masked or muted as in the 'silent' myocardial infarct, when the patient experiences no precordial pain or it is so slight as not to be mentioned spontaneously by the patient or dismissed as 'indigestion'.

Almost any illness in older patients may present in a non-specific fashion with mental confusion, falls, reduced mobility and/or incontinence. These manifestations of illness constitute the common denominators of disease presentation in old age.

Non-reporting of Disease and Disability in Old Age

Another phenomenon which complicates the medicine of old age is non-reporting. In young and middle-aged patients the onset of painful, distressing and disabling conditions will generally lead the patient to seek medical advice, since these conditions may interfere with the ability to be gainfully employed (in both sexes) and the capacity to be an effective mother and household manager (in the case of females). These incentives to seek medical help are absent or less imperative in old age, when there is no job to worry about and the female patient has been widowed and has only herself to care for and the pension comes in regularly whether the person is fit or unfit. There is much evidence to suggest that some of this failure is due to a fatalistic approach which many old people have towards their disabilities. It appears that they may be rather selective in this respect since conditions affecting the respiratory, cardiac and nervous systems tend to be well reported while those affecting joints, feet and bladder are not. Dementia by its very nature would be expected to be poorly reported since the patient often loses insight at an early stage and thus cannot understand what is happening to him or her. It seems that old people have their own ideas as to what the doctor ought to know about and if suffering from painful, stiff knees, painful feet or minor-to-moderate stress incontinence or prostatism, they may well not bother to tell their general practitioner about these troublesome, limiting and sometimes humiliating conditions.

The practical implication is that history taking and clinical examination have to be thorough which, of course, is time consuming and thus presents problems for the busy general practitioner. The question of preventive action through some form of screening or case finding is also to be considered and we have included a chapter on this theme.

BEHAVIOURAL AND ENVIRONMENTAL FACTORS

The effect of some environmental stress upon the elderly is readily apparent, e.g. the aged person whose thermal perception and thermoregulatory processes are defective is in clear danger of hypothermia if exposed to low ambient temperatures (especially if he/she is also receiving tranquillizers or other medication which reduces metabolic rate).

A lifetime of cigarette smoking will lead to reduction in pulmonary and cardiac function and years of sedentary life will reduce exercise tolerance.

These and other factors should be taken into account when making an assessment, and it should always be remembered that even in old age it may be possible to improve fitness by encouraging a healthier life style (as in the Swedish experiment referred to earlier in this chapter).

There are more subtle forms of environmental stress, the results of which may be of considerable importance. Studies of random samples of old people have shown that about 25 per cent have some degree of anxiety state. This is often associated with loneliness, worries about money, fuel bills, etc. and may be aggravated by widowhood or associated physical disability. While stress of this sort may lead to a clearly recognizable state of anxiety, it may in some cases present in the form of somatic symptoms which may then result in drug therapy with all its attendant risks. Common symptoms related to anxiety are headaches, shortness of breath (with overbreathing), lightheadedness (or other vague complaint of giddiness), indigestion and insomnia. Not only will drug therapy divert attention from the underlying cause, but some of the drugs used may produce serious side-effects, e.g. the prescribing of prochlorperazine (Stemetil) for vague unsteadiness carries the considerable risk of parkinsonism, which may then receive treatment in its turn if not recognized as iatrogenic in origin.

Motivation

It is all very well to talk of encouraging healthy life styles in middle and old age, but the fact remains that some old people are lacking in motivation and simply do not want to make the effort. Many such individuals presumably have always been rather passive and inclined to let others fend for them. However, it is well recognized that being placed in a non-stimulating and overprotective setting will often reduce the person's state of arousal and lead to increased dependency. The old-fashioned residential home with its emphasis upon custodial care and its determination to make all the residents fit into the institutionalized life certainly could be relied upon to induce dependency, eventually inducing dependency even in formerly ruggedly independent persons. This is now well recognized by those who run long-stay institutions and every effort is made to offer residents as much autonomy as possible by ensuring that they have maximum say in how they will lead their lives. Similarly the general practitioner may encounter cases where an overprotective daughter or spouse seeks to cocoon the patient by doing everything for him/her thus eroding independence.

Illustrative Cases

Case 1. An 84-year-old widow suffered from parkinsonism and obesity. She lived in a ground-floor flat with her 55-year-old unmarried daughter who had retired prematurely in order to look after her. By day the patient sat in her chair, while the daughter undertook all the household chores plus helping her mother to go to the toilet, to dress, etc. The daughter suffered an influenzal illness and the mother was admitted to the geriatric ward, where very soon she became mobile with a walking frame, able to dress and toilet herself and was indeed fully independent although slow. Her anti-parkinsonian medication had received minor alteration and it was possible, although unlikely, that this was the reason for the improvement. When the daughter had recovered, the patient returned to her care with an arrangement for weekly day-hospital attendance. Only 2 weeks after discharge from the ward she was noted again to be becoming immobile and making little effort to do anything for herself. A week later the daughter asked that day-hospital attendance for her mother be discontinued as it 'only exhausted her'. Four months later the patient was again immobile and dependent in all activities except feeding. The daughter then had to go into hospital for minor surgery and the patient was readmitted. Literally within 24 hours she was again independent although slow. The patient then confided to the nurses that the daughter continually complained of her being so slow and instead of encouraging her to be mobile, she wheeled her around the house in a wheelchair. Despite explanation and cajolery, the daughter resumed her overweening protectiveness saying it was easier and quicker for her, and her mother 'was, after all, nearly 85 years old'.

In a patient who appears lacking in motivation and in whom it seems that this is a new phenomenon then some physical or mental cause must be assiduously sought. This would involve a search for anaemia or malignant disease or a similar insidious and debilitating condition. Another possibility is the onset of depression which is a common occurrence in old age and which may not be associated with the typical symptoms found in younger patients.

The following cases illustrate the complexity of presentation of illness in old age.

Case 2. Miss A. Q., aged 82, was referred to the geriatric service for urgent home assessment with a view to admission. The information from the general practitioner stated that the old lady had fallen occasionally in the past and for the previous 2 days had wandered out of her first-floor flat (where she lived alone), had apparently become lost and confused and had fallen over a dustbin. She had not sustained any injury, but was described as too unsteady and precarious to live alone.

The lady's niece and nephew-in-law were present at the time of the visit and were aggressively anxious that Miss A. Q. should be admitted to hospital immediately. The patient was a nervous woman with a past history of 'breakdowns' in her youth and middle age. She had marked essential tremor, and although a thin, frail-looking person, there was no abnormality to find on physical examination, other than dense bilateral cataracts. Miss A. Q. could barely count fingers at arm's length, and it was obvious, on observing her walking around the flat, that her poor sight was responsible for her unsteadiness, and no doubt for her 'getting lost'. She was orientated in time and place, although she was so easily flustered by questions that it was possible to understand how others had labelled her as 'confused'.

She was already known to the local ophthalmic department and was on the waiting list for cataract surgery. She and her relatives had been told that she would have to wait for another 6 months. Discussion of her urgent problem with the surgeon and the promise of a bed in the geriatric assessment unit postoperatively secured an admission date 2 weeks later. During the intervening period, Miss A. Q. was supported by increased home-help cover and by her reluctant, though caring, niece. Her operation was successful, and she spent 3 weeks undergoing rehabilitation in the geriatric unit, mainly relearning those activities of daily living which her poor sight had compromised, before her final discharge home.

This case demonstrates the need to identify the underlying cause of, in this case, unsteadiness, falls and apparent confusion, which may be obvious but overlooked, and the need to manage the cause in a logical way. Had Miss A. Q. been admitted elsewhere, without identification of her poor sight, she may well have become acutely confused by the move and her mobility may have further deteriorated, jeopardizing her eventual return home.

Case 3. Miss M. F., aged 89, was referred by her general practitioner for assessment of her suitability to move into residential care. She lived alone, in a small ground-floor flat, supported by daily home help and regular visits by neighbours. Her closest relative was a great niece, and there was a family history of unspecified psychiatric illness. She had sustained a mild right hemiparesis 5 years earlier and had suffered from congestive cardiac failure for which she took regular diuretics and digoxin. In spite of these drugs, her legs were chronically oedematous, and she had had varicose ulceration in the past. She also had a left cataract, osteoarthritis of her lumbar spine, hips and knees, and was moderately obese. Her mobility and ability to care for herself at home had gradually deteriorated. Although very attached to her flat, possessions and independence, she had reluctantly come to the conclusion that she could no longer cope.

At the time of the visit by the geriatrician her main complaints were of 'giddiness' and occasional shortness of breath, even at rest. She was obviously agitated about her future, and admitted to a poor sleep pattern with early morning wakening. Her appetite had deteriorated, and she was worried lest she had cancer.

She was mentally alert, and apart from obesity, cataract, osteoarthritic changes in her hands, hips and knees, and non-pitting oedema of both legs, there was little of note to find on examination. She did not have a significant postural drop in her blood pressure, although she complained of light-headedness on walking.

An arrangement was made for her to attend the geriatric day hospital for further assessment—particular attention was to have been paid to a possible diagnosis of depression. However, 2 days later she was admitted to the local poisons unit, having tried to gas herself. Following psychiatric assessment, antidepressant treatment was commenced, although the psychiatrist felt that she was suffering from a reactive depression secondary to her deteriorating function and uncertain future.

She was transferred to the geriatric assessment unit and appeared happy and settled until a suggestion was made that she should return home. She again complained of giddiness and shortness of breath, although nothing was found on examination to account for the symptoms. It was considered that they were due to anxiety. She had several similar, short-lived episodes and on one occasion was noted to be cyanosed and disorientated. An arterial blood gas taken at that time revealed moderate hypoxia and normocapnia. Examination of her cardiovascular and respiratory systems remained unremarkable apart from a sinus tachycardia, and a chest X-ray and ECG were essentially normal. A lung scan, however, showed numerous defects diagnostic of multiple pulmonary emboli. Miss M. F. was anticoagulated and had no further such episodes.

Visits to her home with the occupational therapist confirmed her need for residential accommodation, and she was moved to a local authority home 3 months later into which she settled well.

This case illustrates the overlap between physical and mental pathology, deteriorating function, and the reaction of an individual to life events. It also shows how difficult it can be to diagnose thrombo-embolic disease in an old person. The vigour with which one would pursue its investigation would obviously depend to a certain extent on the intention to treat. This old lady had several longstanding problems, one of which was chronic leg oedema, which made an underlying deep venous thrombosis almost impossible to detect by ordinary clinical means. The symptoms which were due to pulmonary emboli—agitation, giddiness and dyspnoea—can easily be mistaken for those of an anxiety state secondary to circumstances, particularly in view of the attempt at suicide.

SUMMARY AND CONCLUSION

From the foregoing it will be clear that the assessment of need in old age is a complex and often difficult process.

It is important to realize that modern research has shown that function may be maintained much longer than is suggested in *Fig.* 1.2, and when the age decline starts it is generally less steep and more 'benign' than previously believed.

Although age itself is often a poor predictor of need, it is never-theless true that the increasing numbers of very old people mean that a proportion are surviving with very low functional reserves in one or more systems. They have thus survived into a state of minimal reserves and are moving towards the theoretical state of zero reserves

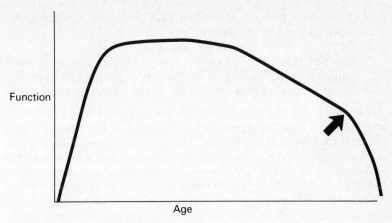

Fig. 1.8. Function and age: the four phases.

in which every organ is working at or near its capacity simply to enable the patient to survive in a resting state.

Figure 1.8 shows the true relationship of function and age in the light of what has been said above.

This figure shows the rapid increase in function which occurs with growth, the period of maintenance of function during maturity and the gentle decline with senescence. The end of this phase is marked by an arrow after which the descent is much steeper representing the fourth phase which we have called *late senescence*. It is the survival of increasing numbers into this phase which is now bearing heavily upon health and social services and future increases mean that general practitioners will be much involved in their management. These individuals have special needs in much the same way as infants and young children—and for similar reasons, viz. their very low functional reserves. They live in an increasingly precarious state in which any stress may produce serious disturbance which may result in system or organ failure which, in turn, may lead (in a domino fashion) to failure of other organs. Homeostasis is readily disturbed, the deviation from normal may be large and it may be difficult to restabilize.

This is by no means merely a theoretical matter, since doctors must understand these matters if a rational approach to assessment and management of patients is to be achieved.

Stress such as relatively minor infection or injury in such patients may be associated with one of the following three results:

1. The patient may die and in some circumstances this may be the most desirable outcome—a short illness with a dignified end surrounded by family members would certainly be welcomed by

many aged persons who often have reached a healthy philo-
sophical approach to these matters.

2. Recovery, which is at any age a satisfactory outcome.
3. Survival but at a lower level of independence. This is the worst
   outcome for patients, their families, their doctors and those who
   have to provide the money for the services they now require.

The good general practitioner has an important role in all these
eventualities. For the patient who dies there is the need for good
medical care and understanding. There is also the need for suitable
advice and support for the bereaved relatives, especially if there is a
widowed spouse. The patient who makes a full recovery does so
partly because of the skill and knowledge of his/her medical attendant
especially in ensuring prompt, expert treatment and in careful use of
any medication which is required. The general practitioner's role in
relation to result (3) above is mainly to minimize its occurrence
through effective treatment and rehabilitation, including early
referral to the local geriatric service for specialized care where
indicated.

From what has been written above, it will be apparent that there is
a very special demand for speed in dealing with the needs of patients
who have got to the stage of 'minimal reserves'. If things start to go
amiss, they are apt to do so very rapidly and if treatment is required it
should be available at once. We teach our students that all need in old
age is a matter of urgency—there is no such thing as a non-urgent
problem. This, of course, runs counter to generally accepted wisdom
which tends to be that old ladies who become confused or 'go off their
legs' need meals-on-wheels or a home help! While they may require
these services, there is also a need for an immediate skilled clinical
diagnosis, treatment and rehabilitation.

The necessity for speed in meeting the needs of relatives is often
equally urgent, since a daughter who is coping with her own part-time
job, and looking after her household and family, has only a limited
reserve of physical and emotional resources. The strain of travelling
to and from her mother's house in the evenings and weekends plus
the anxiety and guilt associated with an ailing mother may rapidly
lead to exhaustion and collapse of support previously willingly given.
Again a rapid and understanding approach is called for.

Looked at in this way, it will be apparent that the traditional
division of health services into 'acute' and 'chronic' is inappropriate
for these categories of old people, since they need urgent care
although not suffering from conditions which the traditional system
would recognize as 'acute'. It is in this area that an efficient geriatric
service can cooperate most effectively alongside general practitioners
and their primary care colleagues.

2 MENTAL CONFUSION

This is one of the commonest manifestations of illness in old age. About 40 per cent of patients referred by general practitioners to the Department of Geriatric Medicine at the City Hospital, Edinburgh, are confused when first seen.

Despite its frequent occurrence and its serious implications for patients and carers, confusion is generally poorly understood. A recent study in an American teaching hospital revealed that, of patients with definite evidence of cognitive impairment, only about 20 per cent had been recognized as such by the hospital physicians. Two of our medical students did a similar survey of elderly patients in acute medical wards in Edinburgh and found that in most patients with cognitive impairment it had not been recognized by the ward medical staff. We find also that general practitioners frequently seem to treat confusion as a diagnosis, whereas it is merely a manifestation of underlying illness. Such a patient was referred as follows: 'Very confused. Going downhill very rapidly. Family can no longer cope. ? Admission.' While it would be unfair to deduce from these statements that the general practitioner had not thought of trying to identify the cause of the confusion, it does seem as though the diagnostic effort was minimal or misdirected.

This is disappointing and rather puzzling, since in many cases careful history taking and observation will suggest a diagnosis (although in a minority of cases this may be very difficult to elucidate and may tax the skill of the most experienced physician). A possible reason for this rather poor performance is the nature of confusion itself, since the patient may be unable to give a coherent account, may be restless or aggressive and noisy and may be surrounded by puzzled, frightened, anxious and even angry relatives demanding loudly that 'something must be done'. Confronted by such a scenario, the general practitioner may scarcely know where to start and may be excused for what appear to be rather feeble referral data.

THE NATURE OF CONFUSION

There are many synonyms for acute confusion none of which add clarity. These include delirium, acute brain syndrome, acute brain failure, toxic confusional state, acute organic syndrome and many others.

Confusion is characterized by impairment of thinking, of recent memory and of orientation. The patient tends to be out of touch with his/her environment and may misinterpret stimuli, thus experiencing auditory and visual hallucinations, e.g. thinking that an incidental noise is a threat to themselves or that shadows in the room represent lurking and threatening figures. Hence the patient may be fearful and respond aggressively by striking out at imagined harmful objects or persons. The state of arousal may fluctuate from time to time with periods of drowsiness succeeded by periods of excitation, restlessness and wakefulness. A most characteristic feature of acute confusion is that in the midst of severe and obvious disturbance, the patient may suddenly appear entirely normal and be able to recognize individuals and discuss affairs quite rationally.

Illustrative Cases

Case 1. The geriatrician was asked to see an 83-year-old married man. Referral data included: 'Recently very confused and disturbed. Chronic constipation, received enema from community nurse 48 hours ago.'

This patient was visited at home shortly afterwards by the geriatrician at 10 a.m. His wife said that he had lately been fairly well apart from his constipation and known diverticular disease. Two days earlier he had received an enema with modest result and 36 hours afterwards during the night he had become very confused and insisted on getting out of bed. Thereafter, he spent nearly all the night in a small cupboard off his bedroom under the impression that he was in his garden greenhouse tending his plants. He appeared to be struggling with an attacker and later said that this was a black man who was trying to steal his plants. When he saw the geriatrician he immediately recognized him, asked how he was, how long he had been in his present post, etc. and seemed entirely normal in orientation and memory. The only clinical finding was diminished touch and pain sense below the knees with absent ankle and knee jerks. He was admitted to hospital where he immediately became extremely confused, noisy and violent. He had to be forcibly restrained by several strong males until an intramuscular injection of 100 mg of chlorpromazine produced peacefulness. He had a polymorph leucocytosis, was apyrexial and had normal chest X-ray and sterile urine. A provisional diagnosis of ruptured colonic diverticulum was made (but never proved). He was given ampicillin and flucloxacillin by intramuscular injection, and after a further day or two of fluctuating levels of confusion he became, and remained, an entirely normal and intelligent old man. He was found to have mild non-insulin-dependent diabetes which explained the neurological findings described.

Case 2. A 78-year-old man living alone in a second-floor flat was healthy and independent. He was well known and liked by his neighbours. Early one morning his neighbours downstairs heard him shouting and were aware of bumps and thumps from the flat above. On entering his room they found him totally confused and almost completely covered by the carpet in his living room. He apparently had got himself under the carpet under the impression that he was getting into bed. In hospital he appeared wildly excited and afraid, was aggressive and noisily shouting. Despite this, he knew he was in hospital and recognized members of his family, knew where they lived, etc. He had a pneumonia which responded to antibiotics and within 36 hours he was mentally normal but with no recollection of the preceding events.

It is by no means invariable that the patient will present in such a florid and excited state. Some patients may in fact be quite the opposite, showing a lifeless and inert appearance or semi-stupor.

Case 3. An 81-year-old single, retired children's nurse was referred with 'Faecal incontinence, confusion and forgetfulness'. She was visited by the geriatrician in her well-appointed sheltered housing apartment. There was a smell of faeces and furniture, etc. was smeared with faecal material. She was quiet and withdrawn and seemed to be confused and disorientated. It was difficult to be sure of her degree of orientation because when asked what year it was she just said: 'I don't know.' A similar negative response was obtained to other questions about her age, address, etc. Her niece explained that she had become more and more confused over a period of months during which she got up at odd times at night, phoned people at dead of night and was increasingly unable to cope. She had a stiff arthritic right knee, was unsteady on standing with a systolic drop in blood pressure of 45 mmHg on rising from a supine position. She was in sinus rhythm. She was receiving digoxin 0·25 mg daily, which she had been taking for years. In addition she was receiving methyldopa 250 mg q.i.d. (also for years). Her rectum was distended with soft faeces. She attended the day hospital where her rectum was emptied and she regained continence. Her plasma digoxin level was 3·5 μmol/l (upper limit 2·6 μmol/l). Her digoxin and methyldopa were stopped. Within 2 weeks she was back to her usual state of independence, was normotensive and without postural hypotension, and remained in sinus rhythm. At routine survey 3 months later, she was fully independent, continent and going out to shops and for social occasions.

This variability from patient to patient and in the same patient with time can produce perplexing presentations, varying from apparent lucidity to states of apparently total confusion and disorientation with gibberish talk. A patient who in usual life tends to be easily depressed, anxious or suspicious in nature will be more likely to show these traits in exaggerated form when afflicted by a confusional state. The person with impaired hearing will be more likely to misinterpret sounds and voices, and if visual impairment is also present, then this combined sensory deprivation will make it more difficult for the patient to establish accurate contact with the environment. It is well known that the evil process of 'brain-washing' is used in order to break down the morale and resistance of individuals in order to get them to behave uncharacteristically, e.g. by betraying military secrets to an enemy. This is achieved by making the subject exhausted, while exposing him to bewildering and often contradictory stimuli. The elderly patient with a confusional state is in some ways akin to the 'brain-washed' subject, especially when removed from a familiar, reassuring environment and placed amidst the frightening, unfamiliar sights and sounds of an accident and emergency department or an acute medical ward. This has important lessons in the management of confused patients since they require positive assistance in orientation in order to help them to keep in touch with their environment.

CONFUSION AND DEMENTIA

Only a few decades ago confusion, dementia and other mental disturbances were often quite undifferentiated and consigned to such rag bags as 'senility', 'cerebral arteriosclerosis' and 'senile decay'. This clearly indicates that few had even attempted to study the different conditions and identify their distinguishing features.

There is now no excuse for this and it is usually quite easy to separate acute confusion from the chronic confusion of dementia. It is important to remember, however, that demented patients are very prone to confusional episodes which may be superimposed upon their dementia, and so the exact nature of the confusion in an old person, seen for the first time, may be obscure until further information is obtained from reliable witnesses and various investigations have been carried out.

Any person may become confused if exposed to a significant hazard, e.g. after an alcoholic binge or post-concussion. The ageing brain is, however, more easily disturbed in this way so that relatively minor disturbances may produce quite severe brain dysfunction in this age group.

A pure acute confusional state implies that although the function of the brain is clearly grossly disturbed, the brain is structurally normal. At the other end, there are the dementias in which brain structure is altered. In severe cases these changes may be visible to the naked eye on dissection of the brain or on an ante-mortem CT scan, and typical histological changes are also visible on microscopy of brain tissue.

We like to think of this in terms of a hierarchy (*Table* 2.1), extending from structurally normal brain to the gross changes associated with dementia.

This means that an elderly confused patient may be suffering from:

A. Acute confusional state
B. Acute confusion occurring in a patient with previously unrecognized early dementia
C. Established dementia with or without a superimposed confusional state

It is very important to make every effort to determine where the patient's position is in this hierarchy since the prognosis is vastly different for the different categories. For the patient with a pure confusional state full recovery may be expected following treatment of the underlying disease. For the patient with established dementia the best that we may hope for is to stabilize the patient at the level which existed before the superimposed confusional state. For the patient with early ('latent') dementia, previously unrecognized, the greatest urgency exists to deal with the underlying condition provoking the acute confusion, since failure to do so may lead to the patient descending the hierarchy towards category C of established clinical dementia.

Table 2.1. The hierarchy of mental confusion

	Condition of	Result of stress
A	Structurally normal brain	Functional disturbance resulting in acute confusional state—totally reversible
B	Early structural changes of dementia	Functional disturbance resulting in acute confusional state—wholly or partially reversible
C	Advanced structural changes of dementia	Patient clinically demented—irreversible. May present with acute confusion superimposed upon dementia—partially reversible

Illustrative Cases

Case 1. An 82-year-old, unmarried, retired female school teacher lived alone in a pleasant small house in Edinburgh. She was visited regularly by her niece, who was in the habit of taking her out at weekends in her car for a day in the country. The patient had been in good health, apart from some stiffness and pain in her knees due to chronic arthritis for which she took occasional aspirin or paracetamol. She appeared to be in normal mental health. She played bridge moderately well, managed her household tasks and finances efficiently, did her own shopping and catering and remembered to send birthday greetings, etc. to her moderately large range of friends, nieces and nephews.

On a weekend outing with her niece she was involved in a road accident in which she sustained fractures of the right tibia and fibula. She was wearing her seat belt and had no head or whip-lash injury. She had no concussion and remembered the accident clearly without retrograde amnesia. In hospital she had a general anaesthetic and the fractures were successfully reduced and a plaster cast applied. The anaesthetic and postoperative period passed without incident. After some weeks in hospital she was allowed home. Her competence was found to be sadly impaired. She persistently forgot appointments, she appeared disorientated and sometimes got up in the middle of the night and phoned her niece thinking it was day time. Her cooking and house-keeping deteriorated and it became increasingly clear that she could no longer be safely left at home on her own. Mental status testing showed that she was mildly disorientated in time and had significant gaps in recent memory. Full investigation showed no evidence of occult infection, subdural haematoma or any other feature which would satisfactorily explain the deterioration. It seems therefore that she may have belonged to category B above, i.e. with some early changes of dementia, but prior to the accident this was in a completely compensated state. With the accident and its sequelae the compensatory mechanisms were eroded and therefore she progressed to phase C. Scrutiny of the anaesthetist's records and her postoperative course failed to show any episode which might have provided an alternative explanation. Despite every effort, she remained in a precarious state at home where she remained for some time with support from the niece and the home-help service. Within a year, however, she required residential care where she settled after an initial period of increased disorientation and restlessness.

Case 2. Mr J. McK. was a 74-year-old widower who had a past history of resected bronchogenic carcinoma, 13 years previously, and of alcohol abuse. He continued to smoke heavily but drank very little. He lived alone in a ground-floor flat and was well supported by family, friends and his home help. Normally he was mobile outside with a stick, and was known to be a mentally alert, if somewhat eccentric man.

He was referred to the geriatric service with the problems of reduced mobility and confusion. He had become verbally abusive to his home help and his daughter. There was a query whether he should be referred for psychogeriatric assessment, but his poor mobility (he had been chair-bound for a week) and his previous alertness strongly suggested an underlying physical cause for his confusion.

On admission to the geriatric unit he became acutely disturbed. He climbed out of bed and threw a zimmer frame through a nearby window. He was given intramuscular sedation with difficulty and eventually became virtually comatose. Physical examination was unhelpful, but a blood urea was markedly raised at 30 mmol/l (having been normal some months earlier). The biochemical picture suggested dehydration, and it emerged that he had developed acute low-back pain several days earlier for which he had taken large quantities of dihydrocodeine, prescribed many months before. Subsequent X-rays revealed an osteoporotic collapse of the body of the third lumbar vertebra. Mr J. McK. was rehydrated with intravenous fluids, his urea fell to normal and he recovered completely. He remembered his violent outburst and was appalled by it. Further investigation did not unearth any intrinsic renal pathology.

Several points are raised by this presentation. First, old people are particularly vulnerable to drugs and dehydration. Secondly, acute illness often presents as confusion, although rarely in such a violent form. Thirdly, it may be difficult for a general practitioner to know where to refer an acutely disturbed old person, particularly if he is not familiar with the patient's previous mental state. It can be difficult to manage such a person in a medical or geriatric ward, in which there are frail and seriously ill patients. There is a place for a jointly managed geriatric/psychogeriatric assessment unit within a district general hospital, where the different skills of the medical and nursing staff can be used together to great advantage. Such units are regrettably rare.

Less Common Causes of Confusion
We would like to illustrate only two of the less common causes of confusion.

The first is the condition called 'pseudodementia' which is a depressive illness masquerading as dementia and presenting with varying degrees of confusion. In the early stages of dementia, especially when insight is retained, some dementia patients may have an associated depression which should be diagnosed and treated with great care (since the dementing person is prone to adverse drug reactions especially antidepressants with strong anticholinergic effects). Severe depression in an elderly patient may also sometimes cause such a marked disturbance of cognitive function that the patient indeed suffers from a form of secondary dementia. In other cases the form of presentation may lead to misdiagnosis of dementia when the condition is really depression. It will be readily appreciated how important it is to make a correct diagnosis in these circumstances since, once the patients are labelled as 'demented', they are apt to be placed in the category of 'unpopular' patients and receive less enthusiastic support from their medical and nursing attendants.

Certain features may help to identify the depressed patient and separate this condition from primary dementia. By far the most important requirement is an accurate chronological history. The depressed patient is more likely to have a short history of mental disturbance and it may have had a more or less abrupt onset. Thus an old lady who presents with a picture of moderate dementia, but the relatives and others steadfastly maintain that she was functioning normally only three or four months ago, must be assumed to have a secondary form of dementia and depression must be high on the list of possible causes. A previous history of mood disturbance must also be diligently sought and may be quite difficult to obtain since the last overt depression may be 40 or more years previously. Careful observation of the patient and clues from relatives or other carers may yield suggestive evidence. The patient may make self-deprecatory remarks such as: 'You should not be wasting your time on me, nurse, because I'm not worth it.' Likewise the patient may appear withdrawn and detached and during history taking is apt to respond to questions with 'I don't know' rather than give erroneous answers as in dementia. The depressed patient is also usually more distressed by his/her mental state than the demented patient and may give a detailed account of how his/her memory has failed and the problems this has caused. There is little doubt that pseudodementia is underdiagnosed and a good rule is to refer early to the geriatric or psychogeriatric service any demented patient in whom there is the slightest reason to doubt that the condition is not primary. There are good reasons for specialist referral in all cases of dementia. We ourselves certainly prefer to know of these cases early rather than late so that we may help to exclude secondary and potentially treatable conditions and cooperate with the primary care team in a programme of optimum management of the patient and support for the family.

Illustrative Cases

Case 1. A 79-year-old widow lived alone with good support from two daughters who lived nearby. She had severe disability due to longstanding rheumatoid arthritis which affected mainly hands, elbows, shoulders and knees. She could walk slowly with a frame and could just manage to get on and off her bed. She had a special chair with a spring-loaded 'ejector' mechanism and a raised toilet seat. With family support and help from a 70-year-old neighbour and the home-help service she managed well at home. A major problem was that she needed help with dressing and in toileting because of her rheumatoid disabilities. She had always been a strong-willed and independent person. She was referred to the geriatric service after 3 months of increasing confusion and disorientation. During this time she had become less able to manage. She had been much more demanding and complained that her family were not supporting her and that she could not manage at home any longer. The 70-year-old neighbour became involved in greatly increased support and became herself anxious and tired out. On admission to the geriatric unit, she showed patchy memory failure and marked disorientation, sometimes stating that she was back at an address where she had lived years before. The nursing staff reported that she made strange remarks, e.g. that other patients were watching her and that she was in any case 'no good and would be better dead'. An early diagnosis of subacute confusional state gradually was altered to one of depression and she made an eventual recovery with antidepressant therapy, but it was a full 6 weeks before the treatment was effective because in the early stages there was trouble with drug-induced postural hypotension and it was necessary to change the antidepressant.

No reliable history of previous mood disturbance was obtained for this patient. Of interest is the fact that she never managed to get home again, despite the fact that her condition was eventually at least as good as it had been prior to her illness. This was almost certainly because the daughters and the 70-year-old neighbour had been exposed to too much stress and anxiety during the 3 months before the patient was referred, i.e. this was a late referral with the expected result of breakdown in support.

Case 2. Mrs E. H. was a 66-year-old married woman with a history of ischaemic heart disease for which she had undergone coronary artery bypass surgery some 6 months before presenting to the geriatric service. Two weeks prior to presentation she stopped eating, drinking and taking the diuretics which she had used for several years. Unrousable on admission, she was grossly dehydrated with a blood urea of 71 mmol/l. Rehydrated with intravenous fluids, the next few days were complicated by episodes of supraventricular tachycardia, and grand mal fits. Eventually her physical state was satisfactory, but she remained withdrawn and unwilling to eat, drink or take oral medication. It was difficult to assess her mental state as she either would not or could not reply to questions.

In the meantime, it had emerged that Mrs E. H. had behaved in a similar way after her cardiac surgery, and had been 'odd' and 'forgetful' in the intervening 6 months. There was no other past history of psychiatric illness, but there had been longstanding difficulties between Mrs E. H. and her husband, the nature of which suggested that she may have been depressed for several months at a time during her middle age.

A CT scan showed significant cerebral atrophy and it was considered that she probably suffered from Alzheimer-type dementia. Differential diagnosis included brain damage following cardiac surgery or the more recent uraemic episode, and severe retarded depression. She refused to take antidepressant drugs, and there was considerable reluctance to the use of electroconvulsive therapy, in view of her recent medical problems. On the other hand, her refusal to eat was potentially life-threatening, and it was agreed to give a series of electroconvulsive therapy. By the fourth treatment, Mrs E. H. had begun to eat without encouragement, and 2 months later was regarded by her family as being 'back to normal'.

This was a particularly complex case, but underlines the difficulty of differentiating between dementia and depression, and the need, on occasion, for the use of electroconvulsive therapy. The CT scan was repeated some months later in case the severe dehydration had produced artefactual atrophy, but remained unchanged, and apparently abnormal, at a time when Mrs E. H. was intellectually unimpaired.

The other unusual cause of confusion which we shall describe is that associated with withdrawal symptoms. The commonest form is delirium tremens which is the excited confused state occurring in an alcoholic after sudden cessation of intake. This may occur in patients admitted to hospital for any cause in whom a sudden acute confusional state supervenes two or three days later (sometimes postoperatively if there has been emergency surgery). Occasionally it may happen at home as when an old lady has been widowed or had an illness in her own home and is taken into her daughter's home who lives at some distance. Despite a genteel appearance, alcohol-withdrawal symptoms must be suspected if she suddenly becomes confused and distressed a few days later. Telltale signs would be stigmata of alcoholic liver disease, raised mean corpuscular volume and abnormal tests of cellular liver function. In the past severe withdrawal symptoms were common with cessation of barbiturates, but these drugs are much less commonly used now although the dangers of sudden withdrawal must be remembered.

Benzodiazepine withdrawal is now recognized as a considerable danger and this indicates the necessity for great care in prescribing such drugs and a determination to ensure that patients are not given prolonged courses of these drugs except in the most unusual circumstances.

HOW SHOULD THE GENERAL PRACTITIONER ASSESS THE CONFUSED ELDERLY PATIENT?

As in most medical conditions, the most important requirement is an accurate history and the general practitioner has an advantage here over most other doctors, since he may well have known the patient for some time and may possess records going back many years. He may likewise have knowledge of and access to other individuals who can provide him with accurate supporting evidence. In distinguishing confusional states from dementia, the most important requirement is an accurate chronological account of the patient's condition. He must try to establish how long the condition has existed and this may be very difficult since family members may not have consciously observed deviations from normal. Thus it is not uncommon for a husband and wife to be coping well together. The husband dies suddenly and it then appears that the widow is unable to manage and on testing she is found to be significantly demented. Her dementia had been success-fully hidden by her husband and the superficial contacts with the family had not revealed it to them. Specific inquiry should therefore be made as to the patient's general competence over the last few months or years. Was she managing her own affairs, collecting her pension, paying rent and fuel bills; was she doing her own shopping, cooking, etc.? Was she still sending out birthday cards, etc.? If not, when did someone take over these activities and responsibilities? Is there any evidence in the home of lowered standards of house-keeping, cleanliness, tidiness, catering, etc.? How does she look in terms of cleanliness and state of her clothing, her hair style, etc.?

If it can be established that she was coping normally ('normal' in keeping with her age) until a few weeks or months ago, then the chances of an acute or subacute confusional state are increased. It must be remembered that relatives may actually set out to deceive the inquirer and to pretend that everything was all right until just a few weeks ago when mother had a fall or was frightened by a burglar or received a new drug from her general practitioner. Just as with mentally subnormal children, families understandably prefer to believe that someone else or some event is responsible for the condition rather than accept that mother is becoming mentally unwell. Hence it is advisable to seek evidence from as many sources as possible in order to check the history given by those relatives who are most closely involved with the patient.

Causes of Confusion

Dementia is common in old age. About 1 in 10 of persons over the age of 65 have been found to be demented in several population surveys with steep increases to about 1 in 5 of persons over 80. Although many conditions may produce dementia in old age, the great majority are of the Alzheimer type with idiopathic loss of brain tissue, dilatation of ventricles and widened cerebral sulci. The second commonest cause is multi-infarct dementia in which areas of the brain are progressively 'knocked off' by infarction, each producing a sudden deterioration in mental function with only partial recovery towards the previous level of functioning. Perhaps 10–20 per cent of cases are of mixed Alzheimer and multi-infarct type. Acute or subacute confusional states may result from almost any illness in old age. The commonest cause is probably drugs and virtually any drug may lead to confusion. The commonest offenders are anticholinergics (anti-depressants and antiparkinsonian drugs), major and minor tran-quillizers, L-dopa and digitalis preparations. In the presence of a recent onset of confusion current medication must be suspect and a first step would be to review all drugs and stop as many as possible. Any infection may cause confusion, the commonest being respiratory and urinary tract infection although cellulitis or any other infection may have a similar effect. Metabolic disturbances may cause con-fusion as in hyper- or hypoglycaemia, uraemia, hyperuricaemia and hypercalcaemia. Head injury (with or without subdural haematoma) and hypoxic conditions may also lead to confusion, e.g. during a general anaesthetic. Cerebral tumour and stroke may produce confusion but will usually be accompanied by telltale neurological signs. Vitamin-B_{12} deficiency is an uncommon cause of confusion and other nutritional deficiencies such as thiamine may rarely be responsible.

Full physical examination is therefore necessary, although this may be difficult in an acutely confused and disturbed patient.

Blood and urine samples should be obtained for haemoglobin and white-cell count, glycosuria, proteinuria, urea and electrolytes and calcium levels. Cardiac enzymes may usefully be included in this screening since acute myocardial infarction may be the underlying cause.

The Detection of Cognitive Impairment

This is generally quite a simple matter although general practitioners have said to us: 'How can I go asking this old lady who is the Prime Minister when I have known her for the past 25 years? She might think I'm going mad!'

Several simple and effective instruments are available. We routinely use two simple questionnaires. One is the so-called 'set test' in which the patient is asked to name as many objects of certain types as possible. These are (1) towns, (2) colours, (3) fruits and (4) flowers. A normal old person will readily offer ten examples in each category with no repetitions and minimal hesitation. This test affords reproducible results and has the great advantage that it presents no threat to the patient since there is no required level of achievement and it is therefore less distressing than many other tests. The result of the test may be conveniently expressed as $x/40$ where x represents the sum of the patient's achievement. Most old people have no difficulty in scoring 35–40.

The other is the Isaacs–Walkey test (Isaacs and Walkey, 1963).

There are several variants of this memory/orientation test and they are all equally useful.

Other tests which may be used are: (1) asking the patient to repeat a series of 5 or 6 digits and then to count them backwards, (2) giving the patient a fictitious name and address and asking him/her to repeat it until he/she is word perfect, then saying: 'I shall ask you to repeat this name and address later' and exactly 5 minutes later asking him/her to repeat it.

Although the practitioner may feel rather uneasy at asking his patients to perform in this way, the fact is that patients are probably less upset by this than he imagines.

The results of such testing may be greatly enhanced by the observations of others who may be relatives (whose reports may have to be taken with a grain of salt as outlined above), neighbours, home helps and community nurses. Occasionally an observant shopkeeper may furnish helpful information about a patient, having noticed a deterioration in her shopping habits or her skill with money and change for purchases, etc.

Table 2.2. Isaacs–Walkey mental impairment measurement

---

(1)   What is the name of this place?
(2)   What day is it today?
(3)   What month is it?
(4)   What year is it?
(5)   What age are you? (Allow one-year error)
(6)   In what year were you born?
(7)   In what month is your birthday?
(8)   What time is it? (Allow one-hour error)
(9)   How long have you been here? (Allow 25 per cent error)

Scoring
    8–9 No significant impairment
    5–7 Moderate impairment
    0–4 Severe impairment

Management of the Confused Elderly Patient

Whether the patient is suffering from a pure acute confusional state (category A above) or whether the confusion is superimposed upon a dementing condition, certain rules apply in management.

The first is to identify any underlying condition and institute effective treatment. In the case of infections this means the prescribing of a suitable antibiotic. Other aspects of general management are equally important. The retention of the patient in familiar surroundings is highly desirable and whenever possible he/she should be kept at home since removal to hospital and the ensuing disorientating experience may be uncomfortably akin to 'brain-washing'. A well-known face and reassuring voice may be enormously comforting to the confused elderly patient and relatives should be instructed to stay by the patient, to speak reassuringly to him/her and to offer physical contact and reiterated comforting remarks. Relatives must themselves be properly instructed and informed that they have a vitally important role in helping the patient to regain contact with reality and his/her environment. They should also be told that if these measures are adopted the patient may show rapid improvement.

Attention to other details of management are important. Lighting should be subdued and bright points of light avoided. Deep shadows may be misinterpreted as threatening and if possible the light should be rearranged to avoid them. For many confused patients extraneous noise may be heard in an exaggerated and distorted fashion and appear frightening. Hence the patient's room should be kept as quiet as possible. Perhaps we should take a leaf from the older textbooks which recommended spreading straw in the street outside the home of the patient struggling to cope with a 'pneumonic crisis' which was usually an acute delirium!

The use of tranquillizers is sometimes necessary where the patient is very restless and hyperactive with dangers of increasing exhaustion. We would never use benzodiazepines in such circumstances but would recommend thioridazine which may be given as tablets or a syrup. A test dose of no more than 25 mg should be tried because, especially in demented patients, phenothiazines may have an unexpectedly profound effect. The final dose will be arrived at by careful titration but it should rarely exceed 75 mg per day. An intramuscular injection of a phenothiazine may be necessary in severe cases. The duration of tranquillizer therapy should be as short as possible, e.g. 25 mg thrice daily for two or three days, thereafter tapering off. The confusion tends to be worse in the evenings and in this case a larger dose may be given about 16.00 hours. It is necessary to remember that some elderly patients may develop signs of parkinsonism after quite short exposure to phenothiazines and that these extrapyramidal effects may take weeks (or even rarely months) to disappear.

Scrupulous attention must be paid to ensuring adequate fluid intake since the sense of thirst in old age may be diminished by decreased osmoreceptor sensitivity. In a state of confusion this is, of course, more likely to occur. Fluid intake should be measured and every attempt made to secure at least 2 litres in 24 hours. Where possible, urine output should be measured and a low output of dark concentrated urine should be recorded and acted upon.

Relatives should be instructed to see that the patient is given the chance to micturate at intervals of 2–4 hours. Successful and complete emptying of the bladder is much more likely to be achieved if the patient is offered the chance to micturate in his/her own toilet. If anyone doubts the truth of this statement, let the males try passing urine into a bottle while lying in bed and the females try to micturate using a bed pan or sitting on a commode behind a screen in a busy ward.

Skin should be very carefully cared for. Where the patient is restless in bed, sacral or buttock areas may suffer chafing damage especially if the sheets are rough or wrinkled. Pressure areas should be regularly inspected and where tranquillizers have been used, the patient should be turned every 2 hours. The patient may derive great comfort and the tissues be preserved by using a sheepskin in the bed.

As in all elderly patients, constipation may be a problem and careful records of bowel movements should be kept. Faecal impaction is a real danger and severe degrees of this may readily aggravate confusion and dehydration. A rectal examination should be done, although the timing of this is important since it may aggravate the patient's state of excitation. Even when patient, relatives or nursing attendants allege that bowel movements have been satisfactory, this should be confirmed rectally.

Where there is cardiac failure, the most effective treatment should be applied—digoxin where there is rapid atrial fibrillation and powerful diuretics when indicated. When the latter are given, especially parenterally, both patient and relatives should be warned that the ensuing diuresis may result in a brief period of incontinence, but this can be portrayed as a temporary phase only and as an indication of the effectiveness of treatment.

In cases of pneumonia or acute congestive failure (e.g. myocardial infarction) oxygen therapy may counteract the cerebral hypoxia and thereby relieve the confusion.

Management of Dementia

Too often the diagnosis of dementing illness elicits a negative response from doctors and other professionals. There are no drug 'cures' (in spite of claims by some pharmaceutical companies that their products may slow down the process). Considerable sums of money have been invested in the field of research into dementia, and we hope that some real therapeutic intervention will emerge before the end of the century and render the above statement obsolete.

However, there is much that can be done for the dementia sufferer and his/her carer. The disease is progressive and infinitely variable between patients. It is important to identify specific management problems—e.g. night wakefulness, wandering, agitation, depression, paranoid behaviour, antisocial behaviour, incontinence—and treat each appropriately. Thus, the old man who makes sexual advances to his female home help, because of his disinhibited behaviour, may be more appropriately managed by the 'prescription' of a male home help than by that of a phenothiazine drug.

Perhaps more than any other condition, dementia demands the use of the multidisciplinary team, with the carer as a full team member. Nowhere is it more important to avoid demarcation disputes between professionals. Many agencies cope with dementia sufferers—home-help service, residential homes, sheltered housing complexes, for instance—and there is a need for support and training of their personnel. Voluntary organizations have done much to fill the gaps left by the statutory services in terms of providing day care, relief care in the patient's home and a counselling service. The Alzheimer's Disease Society deserves particular mention: a national organization set up to help dementia sufferers and their carers; it has local branches in many parts of the country and can provide the special support which only those who have experienced the stresses of caring can offer. It should be seen as complementing rather than usurping the role of the statutory agencies, and we make a point of giving carers the address of the local branch. We also involve local representatives of the Alzheimer's Disease Society and relatives of dementia sufferers in our general practitioner teaching sessions on dementia, with a positive effect on the attitudes of the general practitioners.

SUMMARY AND CONCLUSION

Mental confusion is one of the commonest responses of the ageing brain to any form of stress. It may pose difficult diagnostic problems for the physician, but effective treatment of the underlying condition combined with sensitive management of the patient during the confusional episode will yield good results in a high proportion of cases.

Expert management of confused patients in their own homes by competent general practitioners, backed by caring relatives and dedicated district nurses, will often be much superior to admission to hospital and lead to more rapid and more complete recovery.

For the patient with established dementia, the advent of a confusional state may constitute a crisis in which expert help is needed. The general practitioner should in these circumstances institute good management as outlined above and seek help from the geriatric or psychogeriatric service. Delays may have very serious consequences since the longer the underlying condition remains untreated and the longer the confusional state persists, the less likely it will be that optimum recovery will be achieved. Likewise, delays in obtaining help may readily result in the relatives deciding they have had enough with the danger that they will withdraw support which is likely to be permanent. We still find that sometimes general practitioners appear not to appreciate the need for early referral in these circumstances.

REFERENCE

Isaacs B. and Walkey F. A. (1963) The assessment of the mental state of elderly hospital patients using a simple questionnaire. *Am. J. Psychiat.* **120**, 173.

SUGGESTED READING

Levy R. and Post F. (eds) (1982) *The Psychiatry of Late Life*. Oxford: Blackwell Scientific Publications.

Mace N. L., Rabins P. V., Castleton B. A. *et al.* (eds) (1986) *The 36-hour Day*.
  London: Hodder & Stoughton (in conjunction with Age Concern England, Bernard
  Sunley House, 60 Pitcairn Road, Mitcham, Surrey CR4 3LL).
Pitt B. (ed.) (1982) *Psychogeriatrics*, 2nd ed. Edinburgh: Churchill Livingstone.

3   FALLS

An old person who starts to have falls must be regarded as being in considerable danger and requiring urgent investigation. There is the obvious danger that the next fall will result in fracture—of vertebral body, wrist, hip or neck of humerus (which are the four fractures strongly associated with osteoporosis). In addition to this danger, there may be serious loss of confidence and where an old person has fallen and lain for a long period on the floor there may be grave loss of morale. We have encountered cases where ruggedly independent old ladies have been so demoralized in this way that they decided to give up their homes and seek residential care. Old people who fall and lie on the floor unable to get up cause their relatives (and neighbours) marked anxiety, associated with feelings of guilt which are often channelled into demands that the patient be put into hospital.

The onset of falls is often an indication of serious underlying disease or associated with adverse drug reaction. The underlying disease may be readily diagnosed and eminently treatable as in anaemia due to gastrointestinal blood loss, or it may be more obscure and sinister as in cases of occult malignancy.

The serious prognostic significance of falls has been emphasized by several investigators. In a Birmingham study, 125 fallers were compared to 125 controls (matched for age and sex and belonging to the same family practice). After 2 months, 11 fallers had died compared to 1 control; the comparable figures at 1 year were 32 and 8 (Wild *et al.*, 1981).

EPIDEMIOLOGY OF FALLS

Falls are common in elderly populations both in the community and in institutions. Sheldon (1948), in his study of old people at home in Wolverhampton, found that 43 per cent of women and 21 per cent of men reported that they had fallen. Exton-Smith (1977) found similar prevalences in old people in the community and he also noted that in

36

women the proportion increased from about one-third in the age group 65–69 to over half in those aged 85 or more. In men the proportions were 13 per cent in the 65–69 age group and 31 per cent in the 80–84 group. Interestingly there was a slight decrease in prevalence of fallers in the 85+ group of men, which tends to suggest the existence of some fit old men who survive into extreme old age and retain unusual biological vigour.

Most falls fortunately do not result in significant injury. Lucht (1971) found that between 14 and 19 per 1000 persons aged 60 or more require treatment after falling in their homes. Other facts are:

1. Females are more liable to fall than males.
2. The great majority (85 per cent) of falls at home occur during daytime, while falls in institutions occur mostly at night (and especially when staff ratios are low and at time of change of shift).
3. Falls are more common in old people who live alone. (It should be noted that almost half the females aged 75 or more lived alone at the time of the UK 1981 census.)
4. Falls resulting in hip fractures mostly occur in living room, bedroom or on stairs.

MECHANISMS AND PATHOPHYSIOLOGY OF FALLS

In the course of evolution, man became a biped. Although this conferred the advantage of freeing the forelimbs for complex tasks and the use of tools, the loss of quadruped status entailed a considerable loss of stability. In the many thousands of years of bipedal existence, man has developed elaborate and efficient mechanisms for his maintenance of posture.

A fall is always due to a failure to adjust to and correct for a displacement of the body. Hence in investigating falls it is essential to determine the nature of the displacement and why it was not successfully corrected. It is obvious that a great displacement as on the football field will usually result in falling even in a young and healthy person, while quite a minor displacement may suffice in an older and less fit individual. The displacement may be due to extrinsic causes as in tripping over an obstacle or being blown over by a sudden gust of wind (not unusual in Edinburgh!) or it may be due to intrinsic causes as in syncope or vertigo.

The mechanisms involved in correcting a displacement are multiple and complex. First, it is necessary to recognize that displacement is occurring; next is the central processing in the brain of information about the displacement and the environment, and finally there is the initiation of motor action to counteract the displacement. Hence peripheral receptors, central processing and motor effectors all combine to provide a range of righting reflexes. Age changes reduce the speed and efficiency of these responses and this may be aggravated by concomitant disease processes. There is a serious danger that once the old person becomes aware of increasing postural instability that less movement and activity will be undertaken so that further deterioration ensues due to disuse and a vicious circle may thus be established. An old person, who is showing unsteadiness of gait and who, for any reason, is confined to bed for even a few days, may thereafter be unable to stand and walk unaided and require lengthy rehabilitation to remobilize. This danger of loss of mobility in the old is certainly not well understood by many people, including members of the medical and allied professions.

Postural Sway and Age

A healthy young adult when asked to stand perfectly still will be able to do so without perceptible sway. Using a simple device called an ataxiameter, it is possible to measure sway in individuals of different ages and sex. The young child whose postural control is still not fully developed will show considerable sway; by the mid-teens this has become negligible and remains so until about age 45 after which sway increases in both sexes, but more markedly in females. By age 80 or 85 it is quite common for women to show marked sway, which is clearly visible even on cursory inspection and some may look for an object to hold onto before even attempting to stand still. These observations relate only to static control, i.e. the control of the stationary subject, and it must be remembered that other mechanisms and nervous pathways are involved in the dynamic control of posture, i.e. control of balance, while the subject is in motion.

Subjects who are liable to fall have been shown to have levels of sway above the average for their age and sex.

Some consideration will now be given to the various organs and mechanisms which are responsible for postural control and the maintenance of balance. All these mechanisms are interlinked within the nervous system where the information relating to preservation of balance is processed and analysed and effector stimuli sent to muscle groups in order to counteract displacements.

Vision

The eyes enable the subject to be aware of the environment and to avoid hazards within it. The power of visual accommodation begins to decline quite early in life as the crystalline lens enlarges and loses elasticity. By the age of 50 years many people have lost the ability to focus clearly on near objects. This is helped by the provision of glasses which, although greatly beneficial in reading small print, produce distortions of vision for more distant objects. It may take some time to get used to new glasses. Special problems exist with bifocal lenses where the lower part of the lens magnifies more power-fully than the upper. This causes problems on stairs as the subject is then guiding himself/herself by using vision through the lower part of the lenses. This leads to uncertainty as to exactly where the next step is and even in an otherwise fit person may lead to missing a step and dangerous falls. Old people using bifocal glasses are at considerable risk and this is increased at the time of any change of lenses. They and their relatives should be specifically warned to be very cautious, especially on stairs, when new glasses are supplied.

It should also be noted that the transparency of the media of the eye is reduced with age so that less light penetrates to the retina. Hence there is need for good lighting conditions as a means towards increasing safety for older persons as well as helping them to enjoy the pleasures of reading.

Cataract is common in old age and difficulties often arise after operation on one eye, since the glasses supplied lead to considerable magnification of the image in that eye so that the two eyes are pro-viding conflicting information. Spherical aberration also occurs as a result of which straight objects appear to be curved. Contact lenses diminish these problems, but many old people do not tolerate them well. The recent development of artificial intraocular lenses has yielded good results.

A most important mechanism in postural control is the neurological linkage of the external ocular muscles to vestibular and propriospinal tracts which convey information about the position of head, neck and limbs both at rest and in movement. This enables the subject to follow moving objects through the process known as 'tracking', an important function in defence and in man's predatory activities.

Proprioception

All synovial joints possess receptor nerve endings which vary in quantity and type depending upon the joint involved. Receptors in foot joints, ankles and knees enable the subject to be aware of the position of the lower limb, while skin receptors on the soles yield information about the nature of the surface on which the subject is standing. This information is relayed to the brain via the posterior columns of the spinal cord.

Wyke (1979) has recently called attention to the importance of mechanoreceptors found in the apophyseal joints of the cervical spine. It is believed that there are two types of these receptors—one which provides continuous 'static information', i.e. information about the position of the neck at rest, and another which relays information while the neck is being moved ('dynamic information'). These receptors send information to the brain via the propriospinal tracts. They relay also to the external ocular muscles and are responsible for several fundamentally important reflexogenic mechanisms concerned with postural control and movements such as walking or running. It is now believed that in evolution from the quadruped state, these cervical mechanoreceptors have come to play an increasingly significant role in man and may now be more important for postural control than the vestibular apparatuses of the internal ear.

It has been shown that degenerative changes occur in these mechanoreceptors as age advances and some seem to disappear. The common (indeed almost universal) occurrence of osteoarthritis of the cervical apophyseal joints will aggravate the resulting loss of efficiency of this mechanism, as may any serious neck damage as in whip-lash injury in road traffic accidents.

Some of the loss of postural control and increased sway in old age are believed to be associated with these changes. It is also possible that they contribute to the development of the characteristic flexed posture of extreme old age in which the subject stands with head forwards and hips and knees flexed with a slow rather shuffling gait with the forefoot barely clearing the floor.

It should be noted that attempts to immobilize the neck by the use of a cervical collar may actually make the patient feel less steady since the input from the dynamic receptors is thereby diminished. Disturbance of cervical receptors may cause symptoms similar to those of vertebrobasilar ischaemia (vertigo, nystagmus, ataxia) and it must therefore be remembered that, while a cervical collar may benefit some patients with genuine vertebrobasilar insufficiency, it could have the opposite effect in cervical receptor disturbance, which is probably a much more common condition.

It is possible that dysfunction of cervical mechanoreceptors is responsible for some of the vague dizziness and lightheadedness which is such a common and distressing complaint in old age. There are no drugs which can benefit this condition.

Vestibular Function in Old Age

The twin systems of semicircular canals and otolith organs which form part of the internal ear send constant signals to the vestibular nuclei. Any head movement leads to a disturbance of the endolymph in these canals and this stimulates the ciliated cells within the ampullae or dilated ends of the canals. These stimuli are conducted via the 8th cranial nerve to the vestibular nuclei. In addition, the utricles contain the otoliths which are stimulated by acceleration of the head, the information being transmitted along the same pathways. The vestibular nuclei perform very important functions as integrating centres for spinal, cerebellar and reticular formation tracts.

The importance of coordination of eye and head movements has already been referred to. This enables the gaze to remain fixed upon an object while the head is moved from side to side or up and down. Normally the two vestibular systems are exactly balanced, each transmitting stimuli of equal intensity and thus the gaze is steady. Whenever one vestibule is impaired or overstimulated, imbalance occurs and the eyes will not remain steady so that nystagmus occurs.

Age changes are known to occur in the semicircular canals and otoliths with the general effect of reduction in receptor efficiency. Disease may also occur, either ischaemic due to atherosclerosis or inflammatory as in labyrinthitis or Ménière's disease. Acute disturbances of this kind will usually be accompanied by nystagmus, nausea, vomiting and rotatory vertigo. Unilateral reduced acuity of hearing with or without tinnitus may also be detected.

If abnormality of the internal ear is suspected (or a lesion in the cerebellopontine angle such as acoustic neuroma), the patient must be carefully examined for nystagmus and for other cranial nerve lesions such as 5th or 7th nerve dysfunction.

Central Coordination of Postural Control Mechanisms

Stimuli from eyes, vestibules and all proprioceptive receptors are assembled in the basal ganglia where they are analysed and integrated. Motor impulses are then dispatched to muscle groups in order to complete the various postural and righting reflexes. It is believed that the principal reason for reduced efficiency of postural control with age can be attributed to a decline in the speed and precision of this central integration and coordination process within the central nervous system. Any disease such as cerebrovascular degeneration may lead to further deterioration in function.

INVESTIGATION OF FALLS

In dealing with patients who have started to fall a systematic approach is essential and, as always, an accurate and full history is the most important single item. This may prove difficult where the patient has a poor memory or where consciousness has been lost or impaired. A special difficulty is that patients may have genuine problems in describing exactly what they felt. Thus they may say that they felt dizzy or giddy and when asked what these terms mean they may admit to a wide range of disturbances from momentarily feeling about to fall, 'blacking out', feeling faint, buzzing in the ears or even a feeling of turning or spinning (or the room spinning) as in true vertigo. It is very important therefore to identify any witnesses and to question them. Any potential witness should also be told what to look for should another fall occur.

Lastly, it should be remembered that patients may unwittingly mislead the inquirer through their attempts to explain to themselves what caused the fall. Thus when asked if he/she had tripped over something, the patient may say: 'I must have tripped' (Isaacs, 1985). This demands considerable skill on the part of the person taking the history and recognition that 'I must have been dizzy' may actually mean 'It would be easier for me to understand if I actually had been dizzy'! Elderly patients also frequently try to be helpful and they may see such statements as aiding the doctor whom they are anxious to please.

Special Points in History Taking and Examination

Medication

It is vitally important to check current (and recent) medication since many drugs increase the liability to fall. The common offenders are diuretics, antidepressants, tranquillizers (major and minor) which all may predispose to postural hypotension (the last may also lead to further sluggishness of righting reflexes through their central depressant effects). Other culpable drugs are hypotensives and, most infuriatingly, drugs such as prochlorperazine (Stemetil, Vertigon) which are frequently given to old people who complain of vague dizziness. These hapless victims thus receive a powerful phenothiazine which can only be of benefit to the rare examples of labyrinthitis, while all the others are liable to the serious and often long-lasting effects of drug-induced parkinsonism.

Experienced general practitioners will know that it is not enough merely to ask what drugs the patient is taking, but medications should be sought out and the patient questioned as to his/her understanding of their use and dosage. In older patients whose vision and memory are impaired compliance may be poor and it may be necessary to enrol some other person as medication supervisor, e.g. a spouse or a daughter.

How, When and Where Did the Fall Occur?

It is important to determine the time and circumstances of the fall. Was it on rising from bed or chair? How long after the night-time sedative did it occur? What was the patient doing at the time of the fall? Was there an extrinsic force as a cause of the displacement? If so, was this force sufficient to explain the fall? Often these questions (like many others in geriatric practice) can best be answered by seeing the patients and relatives in their own homes where most falls occur.

It is important to know if the patient lost consciousness before or after falling. This may be difficult to determine with certainty since patients (and doctors) may use vague terms such as 'blackout' or 'faint' which may or may not mean actual loss of consciousness. In addition patients may again try to be helpful and say: 'I suppose I must have blacked out.' Patients should be asked what they remember about events immediately prior to the fall and whether they actually recollect descending towards the floor. Did they fall forwards, sideways or backwards and did they strike any object on the way down? If so, which part of the patient was struck? How did he/she feel while lying on the floor and how long before he/she felt back to normal? Was he/she able to get off the floor? Any witness should be asked whether the patient lost consciousness or seemed dazed and whether there was any twitching of limbs or grimacing and whether the patient was incontinent. Was the patient pale or flushed? Did anyone feel the patient's pulse? The patient should be asked whether there was any sensation of palpitations or fluttering in the chest prior to the fall or subsequently.

Accompanying Symptoms

Patients should be asked specifically about feelings of unsteadiness—is this constant or episodic and at times of falling? Was there any pain, e.g. angina? Was there any premonition of the fall or any sensations suggestive of epileptic aura? How is the patient's visual acuity and has there been a recent change of glasses? Has there been a recent onset (or increase) of deafness or tinnitus?

Does the patient suffer from any condition which might interfere with righting reflexes such as parkinsonism, arthropathy, hemiplegia or other motor deficit? What is the state of the patient's feet and footwear?

Psychiatric Illness

Most patients with Alzheimer-type dementia retain normal mobility and balance; indeed the unimpaired mobility of the robust patient may lead to great problems of wandering and getting lost. Some Alzheimer patients and many with multi-infarct dementia may have problems with unsteadiness, errors of perception or occasionally a walking dyspraxia in which the ability to use the legs for walking is lost or impaired, although these limbs retain normal motor and sensory function as evidenced by neurological examination. Some severely demented patients also may be so unaware of their environment that ordinary objects in their vicinity, which are innocuous for other people, become hazardous to them.

In geriatric medicine it is important to remember that depression may be a causative factor in the clinical picture and this applies in falls. Inquiry should therefore be made about mood, sleep patterns, appetite and thought content. Any previous history of affective disorder should be sought. In this context it is important to assess the patient's attitude towards the falls. Where marked anxiety has been engendered, this will certainly predispose towards further falls.

Disuse

It is important to determine how active the patient has been up to the occurrence of falls. Has there been a gradual loss of mobility and activity associated with low motivation and disinterest? The old lady who spends nearly all her time in bed or in her chair only moving about to go to the bathroom or kitchen is certainly seriously prejudicing her already-compromised postural stability and if this continues for a long time the deterioration may become irreversible. 'Long time' in this context means days or weeks, certainly not months. Many doctors and other health workers seriously fail to appreciate that once a vicious circle of reduced mobility leading to decreased determination to walk has been established, the point of no return may occur after only a few days of disuse. Even if the immobility has not thus become irrecoverable, lengthy hospital admission and expensive rehabilitation effort by scarce personnel may be squandered in the process.

COMMON CAUSES OF FALLS

Falls with Loss or Alteration of Consciousness

One important condition, commonly underdiagnosed, is *epilepsy*. In the absence of a reliable witness of the episode, diagnosis is often difficult. Suggestive clues are urinary incontinence, evidence of tongue biting (but many old people are edentulous!) and a period of confusion or unusual behaviour after the fall. An abnormal electroencephalogram is helpful but a normal record does not exclude epilepsy. Some geriatricians and neurologists recommend a trial of phenytoin in patients who have unexplained falls which seem to be associated with disturbance of consciousness. Carried out with care, this can cause little harm and where the cause is epilepsy the benefit to the patient is great.

The commonest cause of falls associated with loss of consciousness is interference with cerebral circulation and many conditions may have this effect.

Many *cardiac dysrhythmias* can result in sudden reduction in cardiac output with corresponding reduction in cerebral perfusion and loss of consciousness. This effect is likely to be enhanced in old age because cerebral autoregulation may be inefficient so that the complex compensatory mechanisms which serve to protect and preserve cerebral perfusion are sometimes impaired. Hence falls in blood pressure or cardiac output rapidly lead to cerebral ischaemia. Tachyarrhythmias and bradyarrhythmias may both be implicated as may sick sinus syndrome. Bradycardia may be produced by digoxin or beta-adrenergic blockade. An ordinary 12-channel ECG will elucidate any persistent disturbance of rhythm, but a normal tracing does not exclude arrhythmia as a cause of falls, and 24-hour monitoring should be sought where the history is suggestive, e.g. where the patient has noticed palpitations, feelings of breathlessness or where a witness has observed temporary pallor or felt an irregular pulse. It should be appreciated, however, that many old people, who feel quite well and who have not had falls, may show numerous rhythm abnormalities on a 24-hour recording so their detection by no means proves a causative relationship. If the timing of an observed arrhythmia on the 24-hour record coincides with the patient feeling unwell, then a causal relationship may usually be assumed to exist. High levels of suspicion would also be justified where the record shows periods of asystole, marked bradycardia, frequent multifocal ventricular extrasystoles or frequent supraventricular tachycardia. Where serious doubt exists, a careful trial of an anti-arrhythmic drug is justified and a cardiologist may recommend insertion of a pacemaker.

Illustrative Cases

Case 1. An 82-year-old man was referred because of repeated falls. When visited at home, he seemed well and denied symptoms between his falls which had occurred two or three times in the past month. He was mentally alert and cheerful. Each fall had an identical pattern—they had all occurred while he was on his feet in the house. He had found himself on the floor on each occasion without any idea of how he had got there. After a few minutes he felt quite well and was able to rise to his feet normally. No one had witnessed a fall but he said they only lasted a minute or two. He knew this because the last one occurred just after he had put a piece of bread in the grill to produce toast and when he recovered from his syncopal attack the toast was nicely browned! By good fortune he had a classic Stokes–Adams attack while the geriatrician was in the house, becoming suddenly pale and unconscious without detectable pulse or heart beat. In about a minute, he recovered consciousness, became flushed and after a few minutes of dazedness seemed back to normal. He had a permanent pacemaker inserted with complete success. Not many cases are so neatly and easily solved as this one.

Much more rarely, patients with severe aortic stenosis may suffer falls due to exertional syncope. In these cases the cerebral circulation is suddenly reduced because of the demands from the muscles for more blood, while cardiac output is fixed and cannot be increased. Usually these patients will have other symptoms of aortic stenosis, such as angina and dyspnoea, and characteristic physical signs will be readily discovered.

Loss of consciousness may also occur in cases of carotid sinus syndrome in which it is believed the atheromatous changes in the region of the carotid sinus cause it to become more sensitive, leading to excessive vagal stimulation and marked bradycardia or asystole. A tight, stiff collar may cause this to happen when the head is turned.

Micturition syncope may be more common than is suspected and occur in old men with prostatic obstruction, especially on rising from a warm bed at night and standing straining in the bathroom or toilet. This induces the changes associated with the Valsalva manoeuvre in which the rise in intrathoracic pressure rapidly leads to fall in cardiac output and thus to cerebral ischaemia. Less common are cough syncope and that associated with defaecation. A related syncope is that which occurs in obese, stiff and disabled old people who have to struggle and strain to heave themselves out of bed or chair and in doing so may effect a partial Valsalva manoeuvre.

Transient ischaemic attacks may also cause falls with loss of consciousness if affecting the brain-stem region. Usually other neurological manifestations would be apparent—dysarthria, diplopia, ocular muscle palsies or other cranial or long tract motor signs. Witnesses should be asked if speech was slurred, if the face was asymmetrical or if the limbs appeared to be weak or clumsy.

Case 2. Seventy-nine-year-old Miss J. B. lives in a first-floor flat on her own, supported by her niece, who works as a home help in the mornings and looks in to see her aunt every afternoon. Over the previous 6 months there had been three episodes of sudden falls with a loss of consciousness and slight weakness of the right side, facial weakness and slurred speech. She required assistance to walk for the remainder of the day and had recovered fully by the following morning. After the last episode she had been admitted to hospital and was found to be in congestive cardiac failure. Control of her failure proved difficult and an echocardiograph was carried out. This revealed a left atrial myxoma and it was agreed that her transient ischaemic attacks (TIAs) were due to emboli from the myxoma. She was anticoagulated and over the next 3 months had no further TIAs. Her cardiac failure responded to frusemide and captopril.

Falls without Loss of Consciousness

First to be considered are falls due to tripping or being pushed with resultant excessive displacement. It is self-evident that a frail, poor-sighted, deaf elderly person with slow and imprecise righting reflexes may fall if subjected to quite a minor displacement which would not topple a fitter person. Where the fall has been associated with an environmental hazard, then this should be removed or rendered safe, e.g. trailing light or telephone cord, raised or curled rug edge, awkwardly placed shelves, inappropriate height of bed or chair, etc.

Postural hypotension may lead to falls. In good health blood pressure is maintained within narrow limits irrespective of posture, but in some old people and in some disease states there may occur a significant fall when the subject rises from a supine to an erect posture. Any fall in systolic pressure of 20+ mmHg is defined as postural hypotension and around this level the patient may or may not experience symptoms. Greater degrees of hypotension are more likely to result in symptoms, while in patients whose usual pressures are relatively low, modest postural falls may led to symptoms. Thus the patient whose supine pressures are 180/90 which fall to 160/90 on rising is less likely to feel giddy or lightheaded than the fall from 110/70 to 90/70 experienced by another patient.

Blood pressure is maintained by the action of baroreceptors in the carotids, which respond to decreased pressure by reflex actions which increase cardiac output and simultaneously cause peripheral vaso-constriction. Random samples of old people living in the community have shown a considerable prevalence of postural hypotension as defined above. Thus about 15 per cent of persons aged 65–74 show this phenomenon and almost one-third of the over 75s. Many of these individuals have no symptoms, presumably because their cerebral autoregulation remains substantially intact, and this means that, whatever other organs or tissues may be affected, cerebral perfusion is safeguarded. However, where the postural drop is severe (40 mmHg or more) symptoms are likely and where cerebral auto-regulation is less efficient an even smaller drop may result in symptoms. In mild cases the patient will experience lightheadedness and feelings of unsteadiness on standing up, and in more severe cases there may be spots before the eyes or even dimming of vision which may culminate in a 'blackout'. The patient who gets up precipitately is more likely to be afflicted and more cautious and gradual changes of posture may minimize effects. Aggravating factors are rising from a warm bed or hot bath and recent ingestion of a substantial meal, especially if accompanied by copious alcoholic libations.

The commonest cause of postural hypotension is drug therapy and many commonly prescribed medications may be implicated. Examples are diuretics (which tend to reduce circulating blood volume), phenothiazines, benzodiazepines, antidepressants, beta-adrenergic blockade and, of course, hypotensive drugs. Where no drug can be blamed, the cause is disturbance of autonomic function which may be associated with diabetes or chronic alcohol abuse. Patients with idiopathic parkinsonism may sometimes show trouble-some postural hypotension and drugs used in its treatment likewise are commonly involved (including L-dopa preparations).

Illustrative Case

Mrs A. H. was an 85-year-old widow living alone in a bungalow. She was seen for assessment of her fitness for residential care. The main reason for her being considered for care was that for the past 3 months she had been falling and had lost her confidence in living alone. Her only past medical history of note was of swollen legs for which she had been prescribed frusemide 40 mg daily and slow-K 600 mg t.i.d. On careful history she admitted to feeling lightheaded on changing posture and all of her falls had been while getting out of bed or a chair. Examination revealed moderate oedema of both feet and ankles but no other signs of cardiac failure, and a blood pressure of 140/80 mmHg sitting, falling to 110/60 mmHg standing. Otherwise exami-nation was essentially negative. On stopping her frusemide and advising her to sit with her feet up on a stool, her symptoms of lightheadedness gradually resolved and 2 weeks later her blood pressure was 140/80 mmHg both sitting and standing. She continued to have some dependent oedema but there were no signs of cardiac failure. Her confidence was restored and her need for residential care passed.

Patients with parkinsonism are liable to falls for other reasons, e.g. their shuffling gait means that their feet do not clear the ground and so they are liable to trip. Severe cases show the classic festinant gait in which the centre of gravity is pushed farther and farther forwards until falling prone is inevitable. They are liable to serious injuries of face and head since the protective reflex of the outstretched arm to break the fall is also often impaired.

Painful conditions may likewise predispose to falls through inter-ference with normal righting and postural reflexes. Thus the patient who has painful osteoarthritis of knees and/or hips may have difficulty in correcting a displacement because the sudden movement required causes severe and inhibiting pain. The old person who has fallen and sustained a painful injury is, for similar reasons, more liable to further falls because the pain interferes with correcting and protective reflexes. Where severe deformities of joints exist, e.g. marked genu varus, the patient's centre of gravity may be so altered in relation to his/her base that postural instability is disturbed with increased liability to fall.

One other possible cause should always be kept in mind and that is occult alcohol abuse. Every experienced geriatrician can cite cases of sweet old ladies of impeccable and genteel heritage who keep on falling and injuring themselves at home and yet on admission to hospital for treatment of resultant injury appear to have no significant postural instability. On returning home the falls recur and also the anxiety of relatives and neighbours. Careful but discreet search in the house or a confidential chat with a relative or friend may sometimes uncover a surprising intake of sherry, gin or brandy (or all three!). Sometimes this has arisen as a defence against loneliness and possibly associated depression. Telltale hints are a raised mean corpuscular volume or abnormal liver function tests.

No mention so far has been made of the condition described originally by Sheldon (1960) as *drop attacks*. The patient is described as suddenly dropping to the ground without alteration of consciousness. The patient is thereafter often unable to get up, although if the soles of the feet are placed against the wall it is alleged that this, in some mysterious way, restores normal reflex control and the patient can thereafter rise and walk normally. The full syndrome as described by Sheldon has never been diagnosed by any of the three authors of this book. Moreover, we feel that the use of this term should be discouraged since it is all too easy to assume that in applying this label to a patient's falls we are making a diagnosis, whereas all we are doing is applying a label which means: 'I do not know why this patient has fallen.' The danger thereafter is that detailed inquiry will not be pursued and remediable (or at least manageable) conditions will be undetected.

INVESTIGATION OF THE PATIENT WHO FALLS

The Home

It has already been emphasized that the best place to start the search for an explanation of falls is often the patient's home. This is certainly so where the patient is completely or substantially housebound and the falls have occurred inside the home.

The trained observer will rapidly assimilate the general ambience—cleanliness, orderliness, tidiness, temperature of the lived-in areas, lighting and odours suggesting incontinence. Special attention will be directed towards the existence of hazards—scatter rugs, dog or cat, coffee tables, stools, trailing cords, etc. Bedroom, bathroom and living room deserve attention since most falls resulting in serious fractures occur therein. A quick look in the kitchen will reveal the amount and quality of food in the refrigerator and larder, and it is useful to try to determine how many pots and pans seem to be in regular and recent use. Any telltale spirits or wine bottles should, of course, be noted.

The Patient

In addition to the search for the clinical states outlined above, certain special observations should be made. The patient should be asked to stand up with legs comfortably apart and sway estimated first with the patient's eyes open then closed. During this process the patient should receive a gentle push on the front of the chest to determine the ability to correct for this displacement. This also should be done with eyes open then closed.

The patient should be sat in a chair, then asked to rise, walk across the room, turn around, return to chair and sit down. Each stage should be carefully inspected for evidence of unsteadiness, tendency to bump into or clutch at objects and for abnormality of gait. Common abnormalities of gait are those associated with pain and stiffness of joints (hips and knees especially), hemiplegia or general muscle weakness (as in osteomalacia). Footwear and feet should be inspected and weight-bearing joints examined for deformity, swelling and effusion and the range of movement assessed.

The typical gait of parkinsonism is easily recognized, but minor degrees may be missed although even these may nevertheless contribute to falls and instability. Careful note should therefore be made of facial expression and voice, fine movements of hands, speed of movement (e.g. finger to nose test), ability to initiate and sustain rapid pronation/supination of forearm. The flexed, short-stepping, shuffling gait of parkinsonism is usually easily distinguished from the broad-based *marche à petit pas* of the patient with widespread cerebrovascular disease. The degree of associated arm swinging should be noted while the patient walks.

Simple visual testing should be done using recognition of common objects and ability to read different sizes of print. Hearing should be assessed during the consultation by noting the ease with which the patient was able to comprehend the examiner's questions and to what extent questions had to be repeated and the voice raised. Each ear may be tested by using a tuning fork.

MANAGEMENT OF PATIENTS WHO FALL

As in all medical conditions, the first and most important requirement is accurate diagnosis of the underlying condition (or conditions). Thereafter this (these) should be corrected wherever possible. The withdrawal of a drug causing postural hypotension (or its continuation in a lower dosage) may be all that is required, but a considerable proportion of patients (especially the very elderly) will remain posturally precarious because of irreversible age and disease changes of the kind described above.

Special attention should be paid to the condition of the patient's feet and footwear and a chiropodist should be asked to help if there are painful corns or calluses or onychogryphosis. Where necessary, well-fitting shoes with low heels should be purchased.

The environment should be made as safe as possible. This involves a review of floor coverings, furniture and fittings, lighting, height of cupboards and electricity sockets, and special attention should be paid to stairs (loose stair carpets, poor lighting, absence of handrail). An occupational therapist is expert in environmental safety, and we strongly recommend that, if possible, general practitioners should make an effort at some time to see how she does her home assessment of an elderly patient and selects suitable aids to daily living.

A physiotherapist may also be invaluable in assessing the patient's gait, ability to transfer, etc. The physiotherapist will also advise upon the use of walking aids. This can be a complex matter and it is important not just to offer walking frames indiscriminately to all who have fallen. Where the patient has recently had falls with painful injury and loss of morale and the underlying cause has been identified and rectified (e.g. as in correction of postural hypotension or control of arrhythmia by a pacemaker or drugs), the patient should be encouraged to aim for a normal gait and full unaided mobility. In these circumstances unnecessary dependence upon walking aids should be avoided, although they may be very useful in the early stages both in securing some degree of mobility (and thus putting the reflexes 'through their paces' and in propping up the patient's sagging confidence). It is important, however, that the patient should be constantly told that he/she is going to manage to walk normally and safely without dependence upon mechanical aids. In cases where prolonged and increasing immobility has led to disuse effects, then lengthy periods of treatment by the physiotherapist will be needed, and the skilled therapist will now demonstrate her value in restoring confidence and remotivating the patient.

The physiotherapist may decide to employ certain head and balance exercises (Cooksey–Cawthorne exercises) which are mostly beneficial in vestibular lesions and much less so in central causes of instability. They may, however, serve to overcome the effects of disuse to some extent and certainly will assist in restoring confidence and raising morale.

In many cases the spouse or a daughter of the patient should spend time with the physiotherapist and patient together so that the former may demonstrate just what the patient can and cannot do and so the relatives learn the best ways of helping the patient. Not only is this a direct benefit to the patient but it serves also to allay the relatives' fears and reduce anxiety.

Many old people with permanent loss of stability will require to use some form of walking aid for the rest of their walking lives. The use of a single stick may offer considerable benefit, not only by increasing the area of the patient's base, but also by providing an additional degree of proprioception via the receptors of the arm which holds the stick. This is even more so when a walking frame is provided—in a way a single stick makes the patient a three-legged animal and a frame makes him/her a quadruped!

Lastly, it is vitally important to determine whether the patient can rise from the floor and once again this ability or inability will be analysed in detail by the physiotherapist. Where the patient is unable to do so it is often because he/she sets about it in the wrong way. The correct way is for the patient to roll onto one side, then bend the leg next to the floor. He/she should then attempt to roll onto that knee and bring up the other so that the patient is then kneeling. By crawling, the patient then tries to reach a chair, table or other support and haul himself/herself up preferably onto a chair.

When patients cannot be taught successfully to rise from the fallen position, then consideration should be given to the supply of an electric or electronic alarm which can alert others to the patient's plight. Usually an occupational therapist will be able to advise on this.

Drug Therapy

After this chapter was completed we noticed that we had not alluded to drugs except as *causes* of falls. We are tempted to leave it at that but this would be unfair and incomplete.

It has already been said that no drugs can prevent falls while a host of them may cause falls or increase their likelihood.

There are a few conditions in which drugs may be helpful. These are almost entirely confined to patients with disturbance of labyrinthine function such as Ménière's disease, labyrinthitis and acute vascular disturbances. In these conditions the patient experiences rotatory vertigo, is often nauseated and vomits and usually will have nystagmus. Frequently there will be unilateral deafness and/or tinnitus. In such cases a drug aimed at quelling the input of inappropriate stimuli from the vestibular system may be helpful. Cinnarizine is claimed to have this suppressant effect as has betahistine, but their sedative effects, while perhaps beneficial in the early acute phase, often make them unsuitable for prolonged use. Phenothiazines undoubtedly help to diminish inappropriate stimuli, probably by an effect in the brain stem and prochlorperazine is the most widely used. It has a strong tendency, however, to induce parkinsonian features which may be more dangerous than the condition being treated and may, unfortunately, persist for weeks or even months after the drug is withdrawn.

Vasodilators have not been proved to be of benefit. Diuretics are valuable in Ménière's disease but of no value in any other vertiginous condition. It should be borne in mind that some diuretics, e.g. frusemide and ethacrynic acid, are sometimes ototoxic and therefore may be strongly contraindicated where there is otological disease.

The Family

It has already been emphasized that relatives of old people who have started to fall are frequently very distressed and anxious, especially where injury has occurred and the patient has lain unattended for some time. When this is seen to be occurring and daughters are demanding that 'something must be done', this constitutes a 'geriatric emergency' since the attitude of the carers is now rapidly hardening and may soon change to anger and indignation. Quite often relatives will then refuse to countenance the patient's return home even if effective treatment and rehabilitation have rendered him/her quite safe and freely mobile. All experience suggests strongly that once the relatives have reached this stage it is very difficult (and often impossible) to get them to change their minds. Once again 'there is no such thing as a non-urgent problem when dealing with aged patients'.

SUMMARY AND CONCLUSION

Falls in old age are common, frightening and potentially lethal. When an old lady has started to fall there are many reasons for urgent measures, in addition to the fact that the next one may result in hip fracture which is an expensive and major disaster for any patient. Falls constitute a 'geriatric emergency'.

The cause of falls can usually be elucidated by careful history taking, systematic observation and the use of basic clinical skills. Many causative conditions can be successfully treated and for those who remain permanently posturally unstable much can be done to prevent or minimize the risk of falls.

The patient who falls will usually require assessment, treatment and rehabilitation by several members of the multidisciplinary team.

Special consideration must be given to morale and its restoration both in the patient and in relatives, neighbours, home helps and others who may readily be rendered anxious and guilt-ridden by the patient's tendency to fall.

REFERENCES

Exton-Smith A. N. (1977) Functional consequences of ageing: clinical manifestations. In: *Care of the Elderly: Meeting the Challenge of Dependency* (Exton-Smith A. N. and Grimley Evans J. eds). London: Academic Press.

Isaacs B. (1985) Falls. In: *Practical Geriatric Medicine* (Exton-Smith A. N. and Weksler M. E. eds). Edinburgh: Churchill Livingstone.

Lucht A. (1971) A prospective study of accidental falls and resulting injuries in the home among elderly people. *Acta Socio-med. Scand.* 2, 105.

Sheldon J. H. (1948) *The Social Medicine of Old Age.* London: Oxford University Press.

Sheldon J. H. (1960) On the natural history of falls in old age. *Br. Med. J.* ii, 1685.

Wild D., Nayok U. S. L. and Isaacs B. (1981) Prognosis of falls in old people at home. *J. Epid. Commun. Hlth* 35, No. 3, 200.

Wyke B. (1979) Cervical articular contributions to posture and gait: their relation to senile disequilibrium. *Age and Ageing* 8, 251.

4 IMPAIRED MOBILITY

Mobility is commonly impaired in old age and its assessment is complex and may test the skills of the general practitioner. Diseases which interfere with mobility are common and multiple factors are often involved. In addition, housing, family support and previous life style may be implicated. Motivation is of enormous importance and it is common to find two old people with more or less the same degree of arthritic changes in their knees and yet one is freely mobile and independent while the other is housebound and dependent upon others for basic needs. Factors such as pain threshold, morale and sheer determination clearly may have a major influence upon the resulting degree of disability and dependency.

In her book, *Staying at Home: Helping Elderly People*, Dr Anthea Tinker examined the daily living patterns of a sample of 1310 elderly people who needed help. Half required help with cutting toenails and using public transport while only 7 per cent needed help with dressing and 4 per cent required assistance in getting in and out of bed and going to the lavatory. Although the proportion of persons with mobility problems is small, the large numbers involved in the whole population pose serious problems for those who are responsible for services for the elderly and for their often hard-pressed relatives who still provide the vast bulk of support.

Other studies have shown a progressive curtailment in mobility and independence with increasing age. More than a quarter of those aged over 75 are housebound. In the UK it is noteworthy that eligibility for the valuable mobility allowance is not extended to persons over 65 (although if in receipt of it before that age, the patient is entitled to continue to receive it until age 75). This may represent fiscal sense, but it also seems to imply that old people have a lesser right to get out and about in the estimation of legislators and the social service bureaucracy.

Any reduction in mobility must be regarded as a serious occurrence and it is imperative that the general practitioner treats it as an indication for energetic diagnostic effort. Too often the old person, his/her family and the medical profession (and we include hospital doctors in this criticism) accept reduced mobility as an inevitable consequence of old age and fail to initiate the necessary inquiries and management to reverse it. Any sudden deterioration is of special significance and must be regarded as a manifestation of major dysfunction. Almost any illness may present as 'going off her legs'— myocardial infarction (frequently 'silent' in the elderly), acute infections, perforated peptic ulcer, stroke, adverse drug reaction— immobility may be the only physical sign of the underlying disease condition. The consequences of taking to bed are serious and potentially life-threatening. They include urinary incontinence, faecal stasis (culminating in impaction and incontinence), malnutrition and dehydration, pressure sores (which may occur within hours, given other predisposing conditions such as poor physical state and local ischaemia), flexion contractures, pneumonia, deep venous thrombosis and pulmonary embolism and, of course, increased stress upon carers. In addition, for the elderly patient whose postural stability is already precarious, every day of enforced immobility makes the task of restoring mobility more difficult and prolonged.

We believe that any old person who presents with sudden reduction in mobility requires urgent and immediate assessment, frequently requiring referral to the geriatric service both as a means of establishing the causes, ensuring rehabilitation and offering timely help to family supporters. Each case must be carefully evaluated using the local sources of expertise and support as judged necessary.

A good history taking will usually reveal the diagnosis and simple questions such as 'Why have you taken to bed?', 'Why can't you get up?' and 'What happens when you try to stand up?' are the obvious lead to an understanding and yet are often not asked. Frequently relatives and other witnesses are able to shed light upon the problem.

Broadly there are five main factors associated with impaired mobility: pain on movement, stiffness and 'slowing up', weakness and fatigue, loss of balance (discussed in Chapter 3: 'Falls') and psychiatric causes. In many cases, more than one factor may be involved; for instance, in rheumatoid arthritis, while stiff and painful joints are often an obvious feature, there may be marked muscle weakness and anaemia.

Reduced mobility and consequent increased dependence on others have a profound effect upon the morale of the patient and his/her supporters and it is often difficult to assess the importance of psychological factors in individual cases.

While any illness can reduce mobility, especially in a vulnerable, frail old person, certain conditions merit attention because either they are common or, if less common, they are amenable to specific treatment and if left undiagnosed may lead to significant morbidity.

Common musculoskeletal disorders are the major arthropathies, osteoporosis and related fractures, osteomalacia, Paget's disease, polymyalgia rheumatica and related cranial arteritis. Many neurological conditions may impair mobility and one of the most common is stroke discussed in Chapter 6. Parkinson's disease (both idiopathic and drug induced) is common but often poorly diagnosed in old age and we shall deal with this in some detail. Thyroid disease and anaemia are important causes of morbidity in the elderly and may present as insidious loss of mobility; they are relatively easy to identify by discriminating use of laboratory tests. On the other hand, dementia and depression may be more difficult to detect since they do not possess obvious markers and the doctor may be misled when the patient and the family subscribe to the view that 'It's her age, you know, doctor'.

MUSCULOSKELETAL CAUSES OF REDUCED MOBILITY

About one-third of complaints to general practitioners from persons over 65 are for 'rheumatic' conditions which encompass a heterogeneous group of disorders affecting the musculoskeletal system. The commonest complaints are of pain and stiffness. It is important to distinguish between joint pain, muscle pain and bone pain—it is only too easy to misdiagnose the muscle pain and stiffness of polymyalgia rheumatica as the joint pain and stiffness of rheumatoid arthritis thereby denying the patient the dramatic relief from steroid therapy in the former condition.

Those neglected appendages—the feet—are commonly the cause of impaired mobility due to bunions, corns and calluses as well as arthritic changes in gout and rheumatoid arthritis. In some patients the inability to cut toenails and maintain ordinary foot hygiene may lead to mobility problems sometimes because ordinary shoes cannot be worn. Regular attention from a chiropodist may go a long way to preventing serious foot problems.

Common arthritic conditions are responsible for 44 per cent of all physical disability in old age and may readily result in patients becoming bedfast or housebound (Harris, 1971; Hunt, 1978).

The commonest arthropathy in old age is *osteoarthritis*. Thomson *et al.* (1974) estimated that 72 per cent of elderly arthritic patients suffered from osteoarthritis compared to 13 per cent with rheumatoid disease. In half of the osteoarthritic cases the disability mainly affected the knees and in another quarter other lower limb joints were involved.

Osteoarthritis is generally regarded as a common final manifestation of a variety of conditions—injury, skeletal abnormalities and to some extent ageing itself. Almost all individuals over 65 will show some radiological evidence of joint degeneration but a large proportion are free of symptoms. Osteophyte formation, for example, appears to be virtually a universal occurrence in old age, although it is probably due to 'normal wear and tear' rather than to ageing *per se*. The practical significance of this is that it may be dangerously misleading to conclude that a pain is due to degenerative joint disease demonstrated on X-ray and hence clinical findings must always receive full consideration. Thus it may be difficult to unravel the exact cause of, for instance, back pain when conditions such as osteoporosis or osteomalacia coexist with degenerative spinal changes. Likewise it is important to remember that disease in the hip or lumbar spine may be characterized by referred pain in the region of the knee.

There are two main varieties of osteoarthritis: generalized osteoarthritis, which has a predilection for post-menopausal women, is polyarticular and associated with Heberden's nodes at terminal interphalangeal joints; and secondary osteoarthritis which may affect one or two joints and be related to an old injury or sometimes to a skeletal abnormality such as scoliosis.

Generalized osteoarthritis may resemble rheumatoid disease—both are polyarticular and associated with morning and inactivity stiffness. Osteoarthritis in a single joint may be confused with gout or other crystalline arthropathy.

Laboratory tests are often less helpful in the elderly. The erythrocyte sedimentation rate is frequently over 30 mm in the first hour in elderly patients for vague and non-specific reasons which have little relationship to the musculoskeletal system; rheumatoid factor is found in about 1 in 6 old people without rheumatoid changes; while serum uric acid tends to rise in old age (and may be significantly increased by thiazide diuretics).

If it is decided after full assessment that osteoarthritis is responsible for an old person's pain and stiffness, then appropriate management should be instituted and it is quite wrong to dismiss the patient's complaints on the grounds that 'It's all due to your age'. This can be very demoralizing to an old person who is having much pain and stiffness and who feels his/her independence is seriously threatened.

Where there is a predisposing cause, such as shortening of one leg, a built-up shoe on the affected side may help. While there is no convincing evidence that obesity itself causes osteoarthritis, weight reduction frequently provides symptomatic relief and makes the patient feel fitter with improved exercise tolerance. Physiotherapy is used to improve muscle function around the affected joint, while local treatment, such as heat, icepacks or wax baths, yields benefit. The physiotherapist should teach the patient exercises which can be continued at home, especially since morale is improved by this form of self-help on the part of the patient. Prevention of flexion contractures of hips and knees is of great importance and may necessitate splints or even surgery. The occupational therapist will provide advice on coping with existing disability and furnish aids and appliances to maintain independence. Where rehousing, or other relocation, is sought the occupational therapist should be asked for her views on suitability of premises for the disabled person.

Simple analgesics are the mainstay of drug treatment—paracetamol and non-steroidal anti-inflammatory drugs such as aspirin and the long list of more recent products which pour forth in 'me-too' fashion from the pharmaceutical industry. While these drugs have an important role in many osteoarthritic patients, they all tend to have potentially serious side-effects which are more frequent in old age and likely to be more dangerous. Recent years have seen the withdrawal of several drugs which had been found to cause serious and even fatal complications in older patients in whom plasma concentrations and half-lives tended to be much higher than in younger patients.

Intra-articular steroid injection may bring rapid relief to an acutely inflamed joint, e.g. after twisting an arthritic knee joint. This may enable the patient to become mobile much sooner and thus retain a sense of balance which can easily be lost after even a few days' immobility. Frequent use of intra-articular steroids is dangerous. Steroid injection into locally tender areas around a joint is often very effective and carries less danger of aggravating the degenerative changes.

Joint replacement surgery has been one of the great surgical advances of the past two decades and has brought new hope to many who otherwise would face a miserable and limited future. Where a single joint is affected or is disproportionately worse than others, joint replacement should be considered. Many factors have to be taken into account—the presence of other diseases (especially ischaemic heart disease, cerebrovascular disease and dementia), the expected benefits from the operation and the patient's general state of motivation. It must be remembered that where other joints are affected, surgical replacement of one joint, by greatly increasing activity and mobility, may increase the strain upon other joints with aggravated symptoms.

Hence it may be difficult to judge the appropriateness of any proposed joint replacement and good teamwork is necessary in reaching the correct decision as the two following cases illustrate.

Illustrative Cases

Case 1. Mr J. M. was a 76-year-old retired insurance worker who had retreated to a small coastal town mainly to enjoy the excellent golfing facilities there. As a keen golfer he became distressed when in his early 70s he developed progressive pain and stiffness in his left hip. The picture was complicated by the fact that he had a long history of depressive illness and when his hip started to cause trouble he became morose and housebound, relying increasingly upon his wife for help with personal chores. At this stage he was referred to the geriatric service with a reasonable request for day-hospital attendance. X-rays showed moderate to severe osteoarthritic changes in his left hip. However, he had fairly good hip movement and it was observed that he walked quite well in the day hospital without complaint of pain. The team in the day hospital found it difficult to reach a definite conclusion—he mourned bitterly his inability to play golf yet was singularly unconcerned over his dependence on his wife. Initially it was felt that hip replacement was inappropriate since it seemed unlikely to restore his golfing abilities as a lot of his difficulties appeared to be related to reactive depression. Over a few months with physiotherapy his mobility improved and he once again ventured out of doors. At this stage he complained of increasing hip pain which began to keep him awake at night. The patient at this stage asked to be referred to an orthopaedic surgeon which was agreed to with some misgivings. The surgeon was likewise unsure of the exact origin of the patient's disability. Meetings were held with the surgeon, the patient and his wife and the general practitioner's view was sought. The general practitioner had known the patient and his wife for years and shared the doubts about the advisability of surgery. Eventually, however, hip replacement was carried out, and in the early postoperative phase the misgivings of the team seemed to be confirmed as he developed a troublesome urinary tract infection with an acute confusional state. This responded to treatment and the patient was discharged home. He mobilized well and had no further pain but he still grieved over his inability to play golf, although he was freely mobile in the house and had pain-free nights.

Case 2. Mrs A. McN., a very deaf widow aged 78, had a right hip fracture 3 years previously. The operation was less than fully satisfactory and she was left with some external rotation of the leg and shortening. A raised shoe helped somewhat but she continued to have pain and mobility problems. She lived alone in an isolated and rather unsatisfactory house, but her passionate sense of independence made her determined to carry on there come what may. She had a previous history of ischaemic heart disease and hip surgery was not contemplated. Then she had a stroke with minor right-sided weakness and moderate expressive dysphasia. At this stage she was admitted to the geriatric service. She made some recovery from the stroke but her mobility was poor. She required the help of two persons to rise from her chair and then could manage only a few steps with a Zimmer walking frame. She made little attempt to dress herself and tended to withdraw from staff and patients. Her son and daughter became convinced that all she needed was a hip replacement operation and thereafter she would be able to mobilize and go to live with one of them. The geriatric team, however, were convinced that the disability from the stroke was the main factor in her dependency and, even if she survived an operation, there would be little or no benefit. At this juncture, and 'out of the blue', it was learned that she had been offered a flat in sheltered housing very close to her daughter. On receiving this good news, she cheered up, started to take an interest in things and within a week was walking the length of the physiotherapy department.

This case demonstrates the over-riding importance of psychological factors in recovery. The patient realized that she could not return to her old house, yet dreaded the prospect of being dependent upon others in their home. Communication with her was imperfect because of deafness and dysphasia. The professionals and her family attached too much importance to her physical problems and in the end she was salvaged by the housing department!

One further point should be emphasized about joint replacement surgery. Waiting lists for these operations in the UK can be lengthy and while waiting it is important to continue to support the patient and offer appropriate treatment and support. Would further physio-therapy help? Should the footwear be reviewed? Should the drugs be changed? Waiting lists can have a debilitating effect on everyone— the patient may cancel all social appointments, while the doctor may dismiss her as 'just waiting' and cease to think positively.

The general practitioner, knowing the lengthy wait for some elective surgery, should be honest and not mislead the patient into believing that it will only be a 'few weeks' when it is certain that the delay will be months or years! Orthopaedic surgeons are prepared to allocate extra priority to patients on their lists when things become very difficult and the general practitioner has a duty to represent the patient's case honestly when deterioration occurs as when pain or mobility become much worse.

Rheumatoid arthritis affects all ages and although it generally starts in middle age, more and more patients are surviving into old age when they require special help and support. The occurrence of rheumatoid arthritis in the late 60s or 70s is now known to be relatively common and female preponderance seems less obvious in these late-onset cases. The result is a considerable prevalence in old age.

Rheumatoid arthritis is generally (but not invariably) polyarticular, symmetrical and affects the peripheral joints with constitutional upset and diffuse muscular pains and stiffness, especially in the mornings. There may be weight loss, low fever, muscle weakness and wasting. Normochromic, normocytic anaemia is common and associated gastrointestinal blood loss due to drug therapy may lead to an iron-deficiency picture. Non-articular manifestations include dry eyes and mouth, pleural and pericardial effusions, nerve entrapment (including carpal tunnel syndrome) and neuropathies. Muscle pain and tender-ness may be quite prominent in early cases and lead to confusion with polymyalgia rheumatica (with which there may be genuine overlap).

Cases starting in old age tend to be sudden in onset and carry quite a good prognosis for recovery (in spite of alarmingly high titres of rheumatoid factor). Extra-articular manifestations of the disease are less common.

It can be difficult to be sure of a diagnosis of rheumatoid in old patients and likewise it may be difficult to be certain of the cause for deterioration in an old patient with longstanding rheumatoid disease. Is this deterioration due to exacerbation of rheumatoid disease, to intercurrent illness (especially depression) or is there an iatrogenic factor associated with drug therapy? These questions must be posed.

One serious danger lurks for the unwary and that is the development of an acute septic monoarthritis in the course of chronic rheumatoid disease. This may be misdiagnosed as an acute exacerbation of rheumatoid and treated with anti-inflammatory drugs or, even more dangerously, with intra-articular steroids. Another diagnostic problem is ruptured Baker's cyst which is an extra-articular synovial cyst behind the knee. When it ruptures, it causes sudden firm painful swelling of the calf, easily misdiagnosed as deep venous thrombosis and then inappropriately treated with anticoagulants.

Treatment in rheumatoid arthritis has several aims: suppression of the inflammation, limitation of articular destruction, control of systemic upset and avoidance of complications of the disease (and its treatment) together with preservation of function and independence. As in all chronic diseases, especially in old age, successful management depends upon effective teamwork between patient, family and the various professionals involved. Time must be allocated for explanation to patient and relatives especially when there is a complex regime of drugs with potentially serious side-effects. Although many rheumatoid patients attend specialist clinics (and geriatric departments), the mainstay of their medical care is the primary health care team and the good general practitioner will respond to this challenge by thinking well beyond the prescription of the latest non-steroidal anti-inflammatory drug.

Physiotherapy and occupational therapy play important roles in the management of rheumatoid patients. Exercises can be taught which the patients with help from their relatives can continue at home. Acutely inflamed joints require short periods of rest with correct positioning (and splinting where indicated) to avoid flexion contractures. A pillow placed under an acutely inflamed knee may offer immediate temporary relief but at the disastrous cost of a contracture. General practitioners should ask the advice of the domiciliary physiotherapist when worries arise over threatened contractures. This is such a grave danger that the rheumatologist or geriatrician should be contacted without delay. Once the acute process starts to settle, graduated exercises, standing and walking should commence. The occupational therapist will advise on the best methods of achieving independence and the provision of appropriate aids and appliances.

Many drugs are used in rheumatoid arthritis, the commonest by far being the non-steroidal anti-inflammatory group. All of these have powerful beneficial effects but also carry an alarming risk of adverse reactions, especially bleeding from the gut, dyspepsia, exacerbation or recurrence of peptic ulcer, diarrhoea and renal toxicity. Some also lead to water and sodium retention and this may precipitate cardiac or renal failure (the latter especially in very old and dehydrated patients). They are therefore two-edged weapons and must be used with the greatest discretion. Faecal occult blood tests should be carried out with regular checks on haemoglobin levels.

Antimalarials, penicillamine and gold therapy may occasionally be indicated in acute cases in old age, but they are slow to act and have serious side-effects including renal and marrow toxicity. We would always seek a rheumatologist's opinion before using these drugs.

The place of corticosteroid therapy in rheumatoid arthritis is still debated. Occasionally a small morning dose (2·5–5·0 mg) may greatly relieve troublesome morning stiffness, but long-term use of larger doses is fraught with great dangers in old age.

Cytotoxic and immunosuppressive agents such as cyclophosph-amide and azathioprine are occasionally prescribed for crippling resistant cases but, once again, this is certainly a matter for the specialist in rheumatology.

Intra-articular steroids have a limited place in management of acutely inflamed joints but care must be taken to exclude pyoarthrosis and no more than two or three injections should be made into one joint.

The orthopaedic surgeon has an important role, even in older patients. Synovectomy may relieve pain and stiffness with functional benefits, entrapped nerves may be freed and joint replacement is now commonly performed. The joints usually operated on are hips, knees and interphalangeal joints. Some patients with 'rheumatoid feet' may derive great benefit from excision of metatarsal heads. Where surgery is contemplated, careful assessment is necessary and where the rheumatoid process is deemed to be active, operation should generally be postponed until the disease has been 'cooled' by appropriate medical measures. Rheumatoid patients often have low immune competence and are liable to infections, including infections around prostheses. Collaboration between general practitioner and surgeon is important in ensuring that the patient is in optimal condition prior to surgery.

About one-tenth of sufferers from *gout* develop clinical mani-festations only after their sixtieth birthday, of whom two-thirds are men. In cases first manifesting in old age, hereditary influence is less important and many are associated with thiazide diuretics or myelo-proliferative disorders. Gouty arthritis is characterized by its very acute, sudden onset and the exquisite tenderness of affected joints. Its classic predilection is for the first metatarsophalangeal joints, but it is not uncommon in the knee. The severity of pain, tenderness and inflammation are usually greater than in osteoarthritis. However, osteoarthritic changes may develop in chronic gouty joints so that the two conditions may coexist. Diagnosis may be confirmed by polarizing microscopy of joint fluid obtained by aspiration when the character-istic urate crystals will be seen. Aspiration is usually only practicable when a knee joint is affected. During an acute attack, serum uric acid levels may be normal and hyperuricaemia bears a variable relation-ship to the clinical picture. Treatment of acute gout is by anti-inflammatory medication until the acute phase subsides and thereafter suppressive therapy. Traditionally colchicine was used in a dose of 1·0 mg followed by 0·5 mg till control was achieved (or toxic symptoms of diarrhoea supervened). At present, indomethacin 50 mg t.d.s. is more commonly used. As a suppressor, allopurinol is used to reduce uric acid production and is highly successful in preventing further acute attacks. Allopurinol should not be given during an acute attack as it may actually precipitate such an occurrence. It is not uncommon in old age for gout to present as a chronic low-grade polyarthropathy affecting hands or feet and associated with tophaceous deposits around the affected joints. We have seen patients with this condition who were described as suffering from 'chronic cellulitis' of ankles. These patients may require long-term anti-inflammatory drug therapy as well as allopurinol.

Chondrocalcinosis or *pseudogout* produces a similar although generally less florid clinical picture, being caused by the deposition of crystals of calcium pyrophosphate in the tissues around the joint. X-rays show calcification in joint cartilage—changes which are present in about one-third of those aged 70+ although the great majority are asymptomatic. Clinically the patient presents with acute or subacute arthritis usually lasting from a day to a month and then subsiding spontaneously. Diagnosis is made by examination of joint aspirate which will show pyrophosphate crystals. Treatment is by joint aspiration, analgesics and non-steroidal anti-inflammatory drugs. As always, physiotherapy should be used to maintain muscle strength and retain mobility.

The incidence of *fractures* increases sharply with age, especially in post-menopausal women. By age 80, 25 per cent of females will have sustained at least one fracture, usually of distal radius, hip or neck of humerus. The incidence of hip fractures doubles in each 5-year age group from 65 onwards and there is evidence from Sweden and parts of the UK that hip fractures are increasing by up to 10 per cent per year (when allowing for ageing of the population). The age-related increase in hip fractures is believed to be due to a combination of increased liability to fall and reduced bone strength. Hip fractures are very important because they lead to high rates of mortality in patients who were previously frail. There is also a high risk of increased dependency and immobility as the old lady who was barely mobile before her hip fracture may never walk again after it. These serious problems have led to the development of geriatric orthopaedic units where orthopaedic surgeons and geriatricians work together with nursing staff and therapists in order to ensure the best chance of successful rehabilitation.

Bone mass starts to diminish after about age 35 or 40 and this loss is speeded up in females for the 10 years following the menopause. When the loss of bone becomes excessive so that crush vertebral fractures and other skeletal changes occur, the condition becomes clinically significant as *osteoporosis*. Factors which affect age-related bone mass are numerous. They include: (1) the total amount of bone present at maturity (in turn this is dependent upon sex, heredity, race, nutrition and amount of exercise), (2) the menopause, (3) certain disease conditions such as thyrotoxicosis, conditions associated with disuse (poliomyelitis and stroke) and rheumatoid arthritis. Reduced mobility and steroid therapy both accelerate 'normal' bone loss.

Calcium balance studies in post-menopausal women show negative balances of 20–40 mg per day. This may be slowed or averted by oestrogen therapy in doses usually sufficient to control other menopausal symptoms. It has therefore been suggested that hormone replacement therapy should be offered to women during the 10 years following the menopause. Unfortunately there are several snags: (1) the oestrogen therapy increases the liability to thromboembolic disease (especially in females with a predisposition, e.g. ischaemic heart disease or varicose veins), (2) it increases the risk of cancer of the body of the uterus, (3) it may be associated with escape bleeding per vaginam and in the light of (2) above this may necessitate dilatation and curettage and other investigations. Hence oestrogen replacement therapy, although effective in reducing the post-menopausal osteoporosis, cannot at present be advocated on a wide scale. It should be considered, however, in menopausal females who have no associated risk factors and who are small (therefore with relatively little bone to lose), who are fair-skinned and perhaps in those of Irish or Scottish extraction.

The role of calcium supplementation in osteoporosis is controversial. Some studies suggest that it may partially restore the negative calcium balance. Other workers recommend a diet high in calcium-rich food. It is almost certainly more relevant to attempt to slow down the development of osteoporosis by ensuring adequate calcium intake (preferably dietary) in young and middle-aged women rather than prescribe large doses of proprietary calcium agents to all elderly women who have clinical or radiological evidence of the disease. Until and unless we have much stronger evidence that the latter course (which would have major consequences for the national drug bill) really does alter the natural history of the established osteoporotic state, we shall not prescribe calcium supplements in a routine way to our numerous osteoporotic patients.

Vitamin D will not prevent osteoporosis. Indeed in 'pharmacological' doses, it may aggravate bone loss through its action in increasing bone resorption. Other therapies promoted for the treatment of osteoporosis such as anabolic steroids and fluoride supplements have not so far been shown scientifically to be effective.

The most common fracture associated with osteoporosis is a crush fracture of a lower thoracic or upper lumbar vertebra. This is because the axial skeleton is affected earlier and more severely than the peripheral skeleton. Crush fracture is common after injury—the usual one being a fall backwards onto the bottom (although it may occur after quite trivial injury or none at all). It is characterized by severe back pain radiating anteriorly to chest or abdomen. It may mimic an acute abdomen or occasionally myocardial infarction or dissecting aortic aneurysm. Diagnosis may be suspected by the radiating nature of the pain and marked tenderness on percussion over the affected part of the spinal column. The severity of the pain may be increased by downward pressure upon the head. The pain is commonly intense and leads to total immobility, the patient being afraid to sit up, turn or cough (even sometimes afraid to speak). Adequate analgesia is essential and in the first few days opiates may be necessary. Non-steroidal anti-inflammatory drugs should be used in order to relieve pain and thus allow some spontaneous movement. These patients usually require hospital admission in order to secure optimum analgesia and prevent pressure damage, etc. The patient should be reassured: 'Tomorrow it will be a little better and again the next day.'

Osteomalacia is more easily defined as a disease entity compared to osteoporosis as it is in no sense a manifestation of ageing. It is a generalized disease of bone caused by deficient calcification of the collagen matrix and is associated with vitamin-D deficiency. The principal source of this vitamin is from synthesis in the skin from 7-dehydrocholesterol under the influence of ultraviolet light from the sun. A small amount is obtained in the diet but the average UK dietary intake is low and most individuals are dependent upon sunlight to maintain their vitamin-D status. Hence the housebound elderly are liable to vitamin-D deficiency and even those who get out rather infrequently may deplete their vitamin-D reserves. The fact that the sun never rises above 30° to the horizon in the UK from November to March inclusive also means that much of the essential ultraviolet rays are absorbed in the atmosphere. Thus most of us are dependent upon our 'summer synthesis' to see us through the winter. Hence a poor summer for all plus a limited exposure for the poorly mobile few may mean that significant numbers of old people are moving nearer to depletion. Previous studies have shown osteomalacia in 4 per cent of geriatric patients and as many as 30 per cent of hip fracture patients. Other predisposing factors are malabsorption (e.g. post-gastrectomy), pancreatic insufficiency and long-term anticonvulsant therapy. The vitamin-D deficiency leads to poor calcium absorption and this has the effect of causing proximal myopathy of shoulder and pelvic girdle muscles with pain on movement, weakness and tenderness on pressure.

Osteomalacia is suggested by the existence of risk factors such as lack of sunlight, low dietary intake and evidence of malabsorption. The classic biochemical changes are low plasma calcium and phosphate with raised alkaline phosphatase, but these changes may be absent or minor. Suspicion should lead to referral for specialist advice which will usually involve iliac crest biopsy to show the presence of excessive uncalcified bone matrix (osteoid tissue). Patients who are housebound (or nearly so) and who complain of aches and pains and who have difficulty in rising from a chair or in climbing stairs should be suspected of having osteomalacia.

Treatment is oral calciferol 1·25 mg per day for 2–4 weeks and thereafter tablets of calcium and vitamin D one or two daily for life. The patient begins to feel better quite soon but myopathic symptoms may take several months to show improvement.

Illustrative Case

Mrs J. S. age 72, was referred to the geriatric service with a 3-month history of increasing weakness, leg pains and tenderness of limbs such that even the weight of the bed clothes was uncomfortable. She had become bedfast. For over a year she had had intermittent diarrhoea with soft stools which had proved difficult to flush away. Four years earlier she had had 3 weeks in hospital with a vague abdominal illness which could have been pancreatitis. Serum calcium and phosphate were well below the laboratory's range of normal, alkaline phosphatase was moderately raised and plain abdominal X-ray showed pancreatic calcification. Further investigations confirmed malabsorption. Treatment with pancreatic enzyme supplements, calciferol and calcium resulted in a dramatic reduction in limb pain and tenderness within a week. Two months later the weakness was improving and she was mobile about the house. Full recovery did not occur until 6 months after starting therapy.

Paget's disease affects 2–4 per cent of the elderly population and is believed to be declining in frequency. There are marked geographic variations in prevalence with, for instance, high levels in Lancashire suggesting an environmental factor in its aetiology. There is a combination of excessive bone deposition and resorption which seriously disturbs the process of bony remodelling (which normally ensures that old bone is resorbed and new bone is laid down in an orderly fashion). Bones affected are mainly tibiae, pelvic bones and skull. There may be severe bony pain, paraplegia due to spinal cord damage and deafness due to distortion of the internal auditory canal. More rarely, osteogenic sarcoma may develop in affected bone and, where large quantities of bone are affected, high output cardiac failure may occur. Fortunately, most cases occurring in old age are asymptomatic and it is likely that many old people carry Paget's disease with them to their graves never having been aware of its presence. In its clinically active form it is accompanied by very high alkaline phosphatase levels and increased urinary excretion of hydroxyproline. Modern treatment by calcitonin injections is extremely effective in pain relief and in reversing the effects of bony changes.

Malignant disease may present with impaired mobility which may be associated with non-specific tiredness and lassitude. In some cases, however, there may be non-metastatic effects resulting in neuropathy or myopathy in which the resulting motor weakness predominates.

Polymyalgia rheumatica is fairly common in old age, being about half as frequent as rheumatoid arthritis in the over 70s. The estimates of prevalence vary from 1 to 3 per 1000 in the 70+ population. *Temporal arteritis* (syn. *cranial arteritis*) sometimes underlies the polymyalgic syndrome in which case the prognosis is much graver (especially in relation to retinal artery occlusion and blindness) and treatment becomes a matter of great urgency. Women are more commonly affected than men and some cases are believed to occur in association with occult malignant disease.

The classic presentation of polymyalgia rheumatica is with proximal muscle stiffness, spontaneous pain and tenderness. Typically it affects the shoulder girdle muscles, less commonly the pelvic girdle. Where the diagnosis is suspected, careful inspection of the scalp must be carried out with questions about localized headache and scalp tenderness. Swelling may be seen over superficial cranial arteries which may be tender on palpation. The patient feels unwell; there may be normochromic, normocytic anaemia and depression. The most important confirmatory evidence is a markedly raised erythrocyte sedimentation rate, commonly 100–120 mm in the first hour. However, in 2 per cent of cases the ESR is not elevated. Biopsy of the clinically affected artery should be requested from an ophthalmologist, but delay in starting steroids should never occur while arranging this because blindness may occur at any time in untreated cases, and, in any case, the typical giant-cell arteritic picture will not be obscured by a few days' steroid therapy.

This condition responds dramatically to steroid therapy and substantial dosage should be prescribed initially. Where cranial arteritis is diagnosed or suspected the dose should be 40–60 mg prednisolone daily. This may be gradually reduced over a few weeks to 10–20 mg and then to a maintenance dose of about 10 mg. The dosage must be titrated against the patient's sense of wellbeing and recurrence of myalgic symptoms but, above all, it must be related to ESR readings. Usually it is possible after 6–9 months to reduce the maintenance dose by 1 mg per month, but this must be done with the greatest caution especially in cases where arteritis has been proved. Enteric-coated prednisolone tablets should be prescribed to minimize intestinal complications of therapy. Most patients will require at least 5 mg daily for 18 months to 3 years before complete weaning can occur. About 10 per cent, having been successfully weaned, will later have a relapse of polymyalgia.

In the presteroid era, about 50 per cent of patients with these conditions suffered blindness. Any suspicion of polymyalgia with or without overt arteritis therefore constitutes an emergency and referral to an ophthalmologist or geriatrician is a matter of extreme urgency.

Illustrative Case

Mr H. M., aged 92, was referred to the geriatric service with the following history: '. . . has been remarkably active until the last month . . . complains of severe shoulder pains . . . can hardly get out of bed because of stiffness.' The patient, a mentally alert man, confirmed this story. He had marked tenderness over the shoulder muscles and could not raise his arms above the horizontal. He could barely move in bed. Blood was taken for haemoglobin and ESR, and, on the strength of the clinical picture of polymyalgia rheumatica, prednisolone was immediately given, in a dose of 10 mg q.i.d. The patient was revisited the following day, by which time he was out of bed and feeling dramatically better. The initial ESR was 113 mm in the first hour, and the blood picture was one of a normochromic, normocytic anaemia. The clinical condition and the blood indices returned to normal over the next few weeks, and the steroid dose was stabilized after 3 months at 7·5 mg per day.

NEUROLOGICAL CAUSES OF REDUCED MOBILITY

The commonest neurological disorder in old age is cerebrovascular disease which is dealt with in Chapter 6. The second commonest is Parkinson's disease, and a long way behind come the peripheral neuropathies (mostly diabetic and subacute combined cord degeneration) and motor neurone disease. The latter must be considered in old age and tends to be more chronic with longer survival, hence the prevalence is higher than in younger groups.

James Parkinson described 'the shaking palsy' in 1817. *Parkinson's disease* is now known to be associated with loss of dopamine synthesizing cells in the basal ganglia, especially the substantia nigra. The cause of these pathological changes is unknown but increasingly it is believed that environmental factors are involved. This belief is strongly supported by recent cases among synthetic narcotic abusers who developed acute parkinsonism after injecting impure drugs and at post-mortem showed the typical changes of Parkinson's disease with disappearance of substantia nigra.

There is a fall in brain dopamine levels with age but only when this gets below 20 per cent of normal will clinical signs emerge. This is, however, important since administration of neuroleptics (especially phenothiazines) may cause the levels to fall below the critical 20 per cent with resultant drug-induced parkinsonism. While this will usually recede in a few weeks after the drug is stopped, it may on occasion last much longer—9 months in one case reported by us (Stephen and Williamson, 1984).

It is still quite common for us to come across patients with significant disability due to inappropriate phenothiazine use, especially prochlorperazine, for vague unsteadiness and falls. This was discussed in Chapter 3.

The overall prevalence of Parkinson's disease is about 1 in 1000 but much higher in old age—1 in 200 of the over 70s. Tremor is less common (50 per cent of our series) and usually less severe in elderly sufferers. Bradykinesia and rigidity tend to predominate, patients complaining of slowing up, fatigue and stiffness. A common early complaint is of muscle aches and depression may supervene at any stage. Onset is slow and insidious and the characteristic stooped posture with slow shuffling gait is too easily dismissed as old age (with which it admittedly has a good deal in common). It is one of those conditions which occurs so slowly that it may happen right under the general practitioner's nose without his making the diagnosis. We have found that sometimes the first suspicion of the disease is voiced by a physiotherapist which is not really surprising since physiotherapists are trained to observe movement, posture and coordination.

We feel that a diagnosis of parkinsonism (or suspicion of its existence) should be followed by specialist referral because its assessment is a complex matter requiring multidisciplinary team involvement. In old patients there are often other diseases and treatment has to be chosen with great care and its effects closely monitored. Thereafter the primary care team will resume full supervision of the patient with perhaps day-hospital attendance for a time.

Where speech is severely affected, an interested speech therapist may greatly benefit the patient which makes life easier for relatives since intelligibility may be greatly improved.

The question of when to use drug therapy and which drug is a difficult one to answer and the high hopes of 'cure' by L-dopa have long since been shattered as its longer term failures and serious complications are tragically exposed.

There is still a place for anticholinergic therapy, especially in younger patients and where tremor is prominent and disabling. We would recommend a careful trial of benztropine in such cases but great caution must be exercised with this drug where the patient is over 75 and especially where tests suggest some degree of cognitive impairment. Such patients may become very confused with anticholinergic drug use.

L-Dopa undoubtedly is one of the great therapeutic advances of the late twentieth century, but like most such 'miracles' it is a double-edged weapon and its harmful effects are more common in old patients. The first question to be asked therefore is whether drug treatment is required at all? Thus an 80-year-old lady who has minor bradykinesia and is therefore a little slower in getting out of her chair and going around the house may not be benefited by the little extra speediness she then becomes capable of. Is she going to utilize this extra nimbleness? Probably not; especially if she is rather obese and has arthritic knees and hips and perhaps has some dyspnoea due to cardiopulmonary causes. L-Dopa in such a case would not be justified and should she develop adverse effects the net effect could be considerable harm to the patient.

Where L-dopa is decided upon it is now invariably given in combination with a decarboxylase inhibitor (Madopar or Sinemet). It is now known that less than about 75 mg of this inhibitor is probably scarcely effective, so choice of preparation should be done with this in mind. Our practice is to start with 62·5 mg of Madopar twice daily and increase by 62·5 mg every 5 days watching carefully for side-effects—mainly confusion and postural hypotension. The physiotherapist and occupational therapist make weekly assessments of progress using timed tests of speed and dexterity. When further improvement is slowing down or has ceased, this indicates the appropriate maintenance dose. When a significant adverse reaction occurs, the dose is reduced by one stage and the patient observed for a few more weeks. This titration of dosage against effect and adverse reaction is very readily accomplished in the day hospital where the team is highly trained in this kind of serial assessment. A common maintenance regime is 125 mg on rising, 62·5 mg at midday, 125 mg in evening and perhaps 62·5 mg later at night.

Long-term effects of L-dopa are very serious and consist of loss of effect when the patient suddenly becomes very bradykinetic until the next dose is taken, the 'on–off effect' when there is a bewildering fluctuation from akinesia to good movement or sometimes akathisia in which the patient cannot sit still but fidgets and paces about. Also distressing is the serious dyskinesia causing athetoid writhing movements of limbs and unpleasant sucking and grimacing facial contortions. When considering the use of L-dopa it is useful to reflect that we may be sentencing patients to this fate in a few years' time. Where these side-effects occur, specialist advice should certainly be sought and some benefit may accrue from the use of newer dopaminergic agonists such as bromocriptine or selegiline. These drugs are expensive and require very careful introduction and supervision and have potentially serious side-effects such as postural hypotension, nightmares, hallucinations and confusion.

Amantadine is a useful drug with fewer side-effects, and although it is commonly stated to have only a temporary effect, we have several patients who continue to benefit from it even after several years' use (as shown by significant deterioration when it has been stopped).

It is important in Parkinson's disease to remember that prescription of a drug is only a part of the therapy. These patients are unhappy and fearful and need strong psychological support. Both patients and relatives often have a good deal of knowledge of the disease and may have misguided notions obtained from television or newspapers. This may lead to hopes of 'miracle cures' or despondency about lack of effective therapy. Either way the general practitioner and community nurse have important supportive roles. It is important that other aspects of the patient's (and carer's) health should receive attention. Thus many patients have severe constipation and need help with bulking agents, extra dietary fibre and a laxative. Parkinsonian patients are prone to depression which is difficult to detect because it tends to be buried and obscured by the features of parkinsonism. It is therefore vital that everyone should be on the lookout for significant mood changes and any unexplained deterioration, while it may be due to progression of the disease, should occasion the question: 'Is this possibly associated with depression?' Practitioners are reminded of the existence of the Parkinson's Disease Society which produces helpful leaflets and provides an advisory and support service for sufferers and carers.

Illustrative Case

Mr A. K. was 79 years old with a long history of generalized osteoarthritis. He lived happily with his wife and was a keen breeder of canaries. He was referred to the geriatric service with a story of increasing pain and stiffness in all joints, difficulty in turning in bed, and in getting out of bed and chair, constipation and depression. The general practitioner mentioned his suspicion that parkinsonism was a factor but wished further advice on diagnosis and treatment.

Examination showed bradykinesia with impairment of fine finger movements. There was some difficulty in initiating movements including walking. His posture was slightly stooped and he walked slowly with elbows flexed and his arms showed scarcely any associated movement. He showed limitation of facial expression although a slow smile could break through the flat features. His voice was low volume and a monotone. No spontaneous tremor was observed but could be elicited by gentle mental stress such as 'serial sevens' (subtract 7 from 100, etc.). Rigidity was observed both centrally (head, neck and shoulder muscles) and at elbows and wrists. Cogwheeling was detectable at wrists.

He responded well to L-dopa and day-hospital attendance. Within a few weeks not only was the patient greatly improved in mobility and self-care, but his mood was normal and even the canaries were said to be singing better than ever!

He attended the day hospital for about 2 months and since then has remained under his general practitioner's care.

SUMMARY AND CONCLUSION

Deteriorating mobility in an old person should be regarded as a sign of underlying illness; in itself it is not a diagnosis. The responsible disease may have a direct effect on the musculoskeletal or neurological systems, such as the conditions covered in this chapter, or it may be one of the myriad of diseases which can present 'atypically' in old age. Commonly, more than one pathology is implicated, and physical, psychological and social factors intertwine to complicate the picture.

The consequences of impaired mobility are so serious for the patient and carers that it deserves urgent assessment. Health professionals must avoid sharing the commonly held view that 'It's all you can expect when you get old'.

REFERENCES

Harris A. I. (1971) *Handicapped and Impaired in Great Britain*, Part 1. Social Survey Division, Office of Population Censuses and Surveys. London: HMSO.

Hunt A. (1978) *The Elderly at Home—A Study of People aged 65 and over living in the Community in England in 1976*. Social Survey Division, Office of Population Censuses and Surveys. London: HMSO.

Stephen P. J. and Williamson J. (1984) Drug-induced parkinsonism in the elderly. *Lancet*, **2**, 1082.

Thomson M., Anderson M. and Wood P. H. N. (1974) Locomotor disability, a study of need in an urban community. *Br. J. Prevent. Soc. Med.* **28**, 71.

Tinker A. (1984) *Staying at Home: Helping Elderly People.* Department of Environment. London: HMSO.

ADDITIONAL INFORMATION

Parkinson's Disease Society, 36 Portland Place, London W1N 3DG. Telephone: 01-323 1174.

5   BLADDER AND BOWEL— CONTINENCE AND INCONTINENCE

URINARY INCONTINENCE

The occurrence of incontinence is frequently seen by the patient as a major catastrophe and interpreted as heralding the beginning of the end. For relatives of patients it presents an ominous threat which may lead them to question their ability to cope and continue their caring role.

Despite the serious impact upon patients and relatives, the attitude of doctors and nurses has often in the past been unsatisfactory, the incontinence being dismissed as an inevitable accompaniment of old age or something which will just have to be tolerated. It cannot be emphasized too forcibly that incontinence can never be a diagnosis, only a symptom of some underlying condition. Hence its occurrence calls for urgent investigation so that accurate diagnosis can be established leading to effective treatment and recovery of continence. As we show in this chapter, an accurate diagnosis can very often be made simply by taking a careful history and carrying out a clinical examination well within the scope of the general practitioner. Thereafter, good teamwork between the district nurse and general practitioner will bring about considerable improvement and in many cases complete cure. In order to achieve this desirable outcome however, some knowledge of the physiology of the bladder and micturition and of the pathophysiology of incontinence is essential.

The International Continence Society defines incontinence as 'a condition in which the involuntary loss of urine or faeces is a social or hygienic problem and is objectively demonstrable'.

BLADDER PHYSIOLOGY AND PATHOPHYSIOLOGY OF URINARY INCONTINENCE

The function of the human bladder is to act as a reservoir until the quantity of urine is sufficient to cause the subject to seek the opportunity to micturate.

The bladder consists mainly of two muscles, the detrusor and trigone. The detrusor muscle develops from the ectodermal cloaca. It forms a basketwork of smooth muscle fibres comprising the dome of the bladder and it extends into the posterior part of the urethra in males and forms most of the female urethra. Contraction of the detrusor causes an increase in intravesical pressure which is accompanied by opening of the bladder outlet and micturition. The detrusor is supplied by cholinergic nerves from sacral roots 2–4. These nerves are excitatory and their stimulation leads to contraction. There are also a few inhibitory beta-2 receptors and excitatory alpha-1 receptors. Some fibres of the detrusor extend longitudinally into the urethra and when they contract they cause a shortening of the urethra.

The trigone muscle is derived from the Wolffian ducts and it, the bladder outlet and the lower part of the female urethra are oestrogen sensitive. Oestrogen deficiency is common in old women and may lead to atrophy and undue sensitivity of these structures which are reversible in response to oestrogen-replacement therapy. The trigone is an extension of ureteric smooth muscle lying on the inner surface of the detrusor and joined by the interureteric bar. It forms a triangle between the ureteric orifices and the bladder outlet. It is rich in adrenergic nerve endings. Contraction of the trigone causes funnelling of the bladder outlet which opens the urethra to allow micturition.

In the male there is a concentration of smooth muscle fibres at the bladder neck which forms the internal urethral sphincter, the main function of which is to prevent retrograde flow of semen into the bladder during ejaculation.

The urethra is a distensible tube which produces variable resistance to flow of urine. In the female the urethra is collapsed upon itself in the non-micturating state and cross-sections show it as a mere slit which is angled horizontally in its upper and vertically in its lower halves (assuming the subject to be lying supine). This configuration probably serves to increase the flutter-valve effect in the urethra. The intraurethral pressure is dependent upon surrounding elastic tissue, the smooth muscles of the wall, the surface tension of the urethral mucus and pressure from intramural arteriovenous sinuses plus the effect of the external sphincter. The last is a circular striated muscle which is capable of sustained continuous contraction and is part of the urogenital diaphragm. It is not required to maintain continence as long as the other mechanisms outlined above are intact. It is, however, essential for continence where the internal sphincter is damaged or destroyed as after prostatectomy. It is capable of allowing voluntary cessation of micturition in mid-stream and is also effective in preventing leakage with coughing, sneezing, etc.

Continence is ensured as long as the pressure in the bladder is lower than the urethral resistance pressure.

Effects of Ageing

There appears to be no significant change in the quantity of bladder muscle tissue with age, but there is an increase in the amount of elastic tissue. Hypertrophy of the detrusor is associated with higher intravesical pressures and may lead to trabeculation. This may result in formation of cellules and even diverticula. These abnormal changes may be related to reduction in collagen tissue. Fibrous tissue increases in ageing smooth muscle lead to less efficient contractions. Bladder capacity is reduced and is as low as 250 ml or less in 40 per cent of continent elderly patients. Where there is cerebrovascular disease, bladder capacity may be even lower. Ageing within the central nervous system reduces the effectiveness of cortical control of bladder activity, and the coordination of detrusor and sphincters may become less precise with age changes in the mid-brain.

Nocturia becomes more common in older patients with 50 per cent having to micturate once at night. This trend is exaggerated in males where there is prostatic hypertrophy with overflow obstruction. The ability to reduce renal excretion at night may be impaired thus encouraging nocturia. The bladder outlet and lower urethra in females show atrophic changes associated with reduced oestrogen production and may culminate in senile vaginitis and urethritis. Oestrogen deficiency may likewise diminish the effectiveness of striated muscle contraction around the urethra, leading to reduced capacity to withstand the sudden increases in intravesical pressure associated with coughing and sneezing and resulting sometimes in stress incontinence. The amount of residual urine tends to increase with age.

Neurological Control of Bladder and Micturition

In infancy the bladder operates reflexly. As the bladder fills, stretch receptors in its wall are stimulated and when distension reaches a certain degree the combined stretch stimuli activate a spinal reflex centre in the sacral cord (segments 2–4). The afferent and efferent arcs of this reflex are via the sacral parasympathetic nerves. It was previously believed that this was the entire basis of bladder neurological control, but there are now known to be several higher centres, including one in the pontine area which is necessary to complete bladder emptying and other centres in mid-brain and posterior hypothalamus which are responsible for ensuring that the activity of detrusor, trigone and urethral sphincters all work in harmony to ensure continence and normal micturition. Thus, although in the infant bladder control may appear to be a function of a spinal reflex, the true picture is more complex, and the integrity of the higher centres and of the spinal tracts which convey afferent and efferent stimuli (in spinothalamic and lateral columns respectively) is necessary.

As the young child becomes 'toilet trained' and thus learns to control micturition within socially accepted bounds, the highest centre becomes effective. This is situated in the upper medial part of the frontal lobe in the anterior part of the cingulate gyrus. This centre enables the subject to be aware of the state of fullness of the bladder and it can also inhibit detrusor activity thus making it possible to delay emptying until the occasion is suitable. *Figure* 5.1 shows this diagrammatically.

The detrusor muscle is mainly under the control of cholinergic receptors with some alpha-adrenergic activity, while the reverse applies to the trigone and urethra.

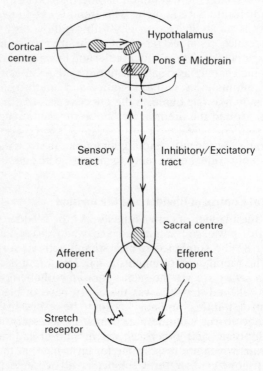

Fig. 5.1. Nerve supply to bladder.

Normal Micturition

The young adult bladder usually can accommodate about 500 ml of urine without discomfort. During filling there are feeble autonomous contractions of the detrusor which are not normally consciously perceived until the combined stimuli from the stretch receptors are sufficiently intense to be passed to the prefrontal centre. At this stage the subject becomes aware of the need to micturate in the near future. Once a convenient occasion arises the efferent loop of the spinal reflex is triggered, the detrusor contracts and the bladder is emptied. The sequence of events is shown in *Table* 5.1.

Table 5.1. Sequence of events in normal micturition

Detrusor contracts Trigone contracts	Involuntary control
↓	
Urogenital diaphragm relaxes Abdominal muscles and diaphragm contract External sphincter relaxes	Voluntary control
↓	
Urine flows, bladder empties External sphincter contracts	Voluntary control
Detrusor and trigone relax	Involuntary control

Although the bladder usually contains up to 500 ml, awareness of the state of distension is commonly felt at 250–300 ml at which time the intravesical pressure will be about 10–15 cm H_2O. Involuntary voiding will take place at about 650–700 ml.

It will be obvious that precise coordination of several mechanisms is essential for continence and this is achieved through the balance between inhibitory influences during filling and excitatory effects at the time of micturition.

Effects of Impairment of Neurological Control

The clinical effect of damage to these neurological control mechanisms depends upon the level at which it occurs.

Where the sacral centre is damaged, an *autonomous neurogenic bladder* will result. Sensation of fullness is lost and the bladder empties incompletely from time to time in an autonomous fashion. This syndrome is uncommon, being associated with tumour or infarct of the sacral segments of the cord.

Where the posterior horn cells or the afferent loop is affected, there is loss of sensation, the effector part of the reflex is not activated and so the bladder becomes overdistended with overflow incontinence. This is diagnosed by finding a distended bladder without the patient's awareness of discomfort. This *atonic neurogenic bladder* was seen previously in tabes dorsalis but today the commonest cause is diabetic neuropathy.

Where there is cord damage above the sacral centre, a *reflex neurogenic bladder* results. This leads to control of the bladder by a simple spinal reflex with automatic emptying when stretch stimuli are triggered. The bladder empties incompletely in this syndrome and the sacral centres are cut off from higher inhibitory, coordination and excitatory influences. Common causes are spinal injury, tumour or infarct.

Where there is damage to the cortical centre in the frontal lobe, the main effect is to lose, partially or completely, the ability to inhibit detrusor contractions. Thus the patient retains awareness of increasing fullness of the bladder but either has only a few minutes before voiding occurs or may be immediately incontinent. This is the *uninhibited neurogenic bladder* which is commonly associated with cerebrovascular disease and/or dementia and is by far the most important bladder disturbance in old age.

Lastly, where the coordination of sphincter relaxation and detrusor contraction is impaired, normal micturition may be lost leading to hesitancy and a poor stream, a condition now known as *detrusor–sphincter dyssynergy*.

Quite often there are mixed lesions as in the *unstable bladder* in which there are elements of both reflex and uninhibited neurogenic bladders.

Another term used is *detrusor instability* which may occur in the absence of neurological disease. In this condition detrusor contractions occur and appear to be unaffected by inhibitory stimuli from higher centres. These contractions may be provoked by coughing, sneezing or changing posture and hence the resulting incontinence is often impossible to distinguish clinically from simple stress incontinence. Further investigation may therefore be required in these cases. Uninhibited contractions may also occur due to excitement or fear, prostatism, pelvic disease, post-prostatectomy fibrosis or acute infection of the bladder. This type of detrusor instability presents with frequency, nocturia, urgency, incontinence and eneuresis.

PREVALENCE OF INCONTINENCE

Various population studies have shown the prevalence of incontinence to be between 4 and 17 per cent for elderly women and between 5 and

11 per cent for men. About 11 per cent of the 85-year-old group will be incontinent. A random sample of persons aged 62–92 in Edinburgh showed severe incontinence in both sexes in 5 per cent and mild incontinence in 20 per cent of males and 37·5 per cent of females. Most cases of mild incontinence in females are associated with *stress incontinence*, defined as 'involuntary loss of urine when the intra-vesical pressure exceeds the maximum urethral pressure in the absence of detrusor contraction'. This is usually due to sneezing, coughing, laughing or physical effort and it is especially common when there is damage to the pelvic floor with descent of the bladder neck below the urogenital diaphragm. *Urge incontinence* is 'the involuntary loss of urine associated with a strong desire to void' and occurs in about 20 per cent of elderly persons.

In residential homes the prevalence of incontinence is up to 20 per cent and over 50 per cent in hospitals for the elderly. Of patients referred to our service by general practitioners, 53 per cent were incontinent at the time of referral.

CLASSIFICATION OF INCONTINENCE

It is helpful to divide incontinence into two varieties:

   a. Transient
   b. Established

a. Transient Incontinence

Inability to get to the toilet in time due to poor mobility or inaccess-ibility, or to slowness in adjusting clothing for micturition should always be regarded as reversible causes of incontinence.

Common causes of transient incontinence are:

   Acute urinary tract infection
   Acute confusional states (*see* Chapter 2)
   Enforced immobility (fracture, other injury, stroke, arthropathy)
   Retention of urine (prostatism, anticholinergic drugs, faecal impaction)
   Iatrogenic causes (too brisk diuresis, oversedation)

While acute urinary tract infections may lead to severe urgency and precipitancy and thus incontinence, chronic urinary tract infection bears no close relationship to incontinence.

Stress incontinence associated with atrophic vaginitis and urethritis due to oestrogen deficiency is reversible with hormone therapy.

Confinement to bed, especially if combined with hospital admission, can readily lead to incontinence, especially if attendants are unaware of the patient's need for regular toileting and the short warning time that many old people have before bladder emptying occurs. In hospital these patients are apt to be catheterized for wholly unnecessary reasons and this may move them one stage away from 'transient' towards 'established' incontinence.

A most important predisposing factor is faecal impaction, often secondary to immobility, poor diet and low fluid intake. The distension of the rectum by a large mass of faeces will occupy quite a lot of the space available in the pelvic cavity to accommodate the bladder and, especially if the latter is already unstable, incontinence is readily produced but remains eminently reversible.

By definition, transient incontinence ought to be reversible, but if left untreated it may merge into established incontinence. In all cases, the longer incontinence is allowed to continue unchecked, the worse it is for the morale of patients and relatives who may eventually simply give up in despair.

b. Established Incontinence

This is almost always due to serious bladder dysfunction, the commonest varieties being:

> Uninhibited neurogenic bladder
> Chronic prostatism
> Urethral stricture
> Chronic retention with overflow (atonic bladder)
> Detrusor instability

Illustrative Case

Mr J. H., aged 90, was referred to the geriatric service because his indwelling catheter was giving trouble. Three months earlier he had presented to the local casualty department with acute urinary retention, which was relieved by catheterization. He was considered, clinically, to have benign prostatic hypertrophy and was felt by the consultant surgeon to be a poor surgical risk for prostatectomy. He was sent home, where he lived alone, with a catheter in situ, and with daily help from the community nurse he coped reasonably well. Unfortunately, after a month his catheter blocked and urine bypassed the tube, with subsequent skin problems. Several changes of catheter were unsuccessful, and on one occasion he became pyrexial, suggesting a septicaemic episode secondary to catheterization. The general practitioner wondered whether Mr J. H. would be able to go on living at home.

Apart from the urinary problem, he was reasonably well. He suffered from osteoarthritis of his hips and knees and walked with a stick. He dressed and washed himself independently, but required help to empty the catheter bag, and his undergarments were continually soiled because of the bypassing of the catheter. He had also developed severe suprapubic discomfort, which was considered to be due to bladder irritation by the retaining catheter balloon.

The volume of water in the balloon was reduced from 30 ml to 10 ml with some relief of symptoms.

In spite of his 90 years, the assessment team considered him to be fit enough to undergo a transurethral resection of prostate. Mr J. H. had initially rejected the offer of surgery, but changed his mind because the catheter was making his life quite miserable. It was important to confirm that Mr J. H.'s main urinary problem was outflow obstruction due to prostatic hypertrophy and that he did not suffer from an unstable bladder (perhaps in addition to the mechanical obstruction). He underwent intravenous urography and cystometry, both of which confirmed simple prostatic hypertrophy. The urological surgeons were happy to operate and Mr J. H. made an uneventful recovery with eventual discharge home.

Age itself is not a contraindication to this procedure, but the preoperative assessment of bladder function is particularly relevant in an elderly population who may have other coexisting causes for incontinence which are not amenable to surgery.

MANAGEMENT OF URINARY INCONTINENCE

Effective management demands full investigation. A careful history should be taken to include questions relating to frequency, nocturia, dysuria, dribbling and urge and stress incontinence. Many women will deny incontinence and yet admit to leaking urine when they cough or sneeze. Presumably they have come to regard this if not as 'normal' then certainly as 'inevitable'. Thus it is important to include such a question at some time in the history taking. The pattern of incontinence should be accurately determined, e.g. continuous dribbling or sudden drenching reflex emptying. Relatives or attendants should be questioned for verification of the history.

Clinical assessment must include mental testing to uncover dementia (*see* Chapter 2), palpation for distended bladder, inspection of external genitalia and, most important, rectal examination.

Urine should be examined for glucose, blood or protein and a mid-stream specimen sent for culture. Obtaining a satisfactory sample in females is achieved by separating the labia, asking the patient to micturate and then inserting a waxed cardboard container into the stream. In males the foreskin should be retracted and the same procedure followed without stopping the stream.

It is useful to devise a simple form of charting of bladder function with timing of micturition and episodes of incontinence. The patient may be capable of doing this, otherwise a relative or attendant should be asked to cooperate.

In patients where history and examination have failed to uncover the cause, the patient should be referred for further investigation, and we recommend that this should be done without delay, both because of the danger that 'transient' incontinence becomes 'established' and the threat to the morale of patient and carers.

To Whom Should the Patient be Referred?

Obviously this depends upon local circumstances and the interests of local consultants. Where there is an efficient geriatric service, elderly patients should be referred there, and many geriatric units now conduct their own urodynamic investigations or have established good contacts with interested urologists or gynaecologists.

The investigations generally carried out are:

a. *Plain radiograph of abdomen:* to reveal urinary calculi and to give an estimation of the state of colonic overloading and stasis
b. *Filling and voiding cystometrogram:* to show the degree of distensibility of the bladder and the occurrence of uninhibited detrusor activity, as well as measurement of bladder pressures at different stages of filling
c. *Urethral pressure profiles*
d. *Patterns of urinary flow*

(Interested readers are referred to excellent texts on these investigations at the end of this chapter.)

The general practitioner may easily detect evidence of senile vaginitis and vaginal smears will confirm the existence of oestrogen deficiency.

Specific Treatment

Treatment of any underlying cause such as faecal impaction, urinary tract infection or the cessation of inappropriate drug therapy is the first line of attack in the incontinent patient.

Explanation of the problem to patient and relatives is always important and this should be done in a matter-of-fact fashion with cautious optimism as to outcome. The accurate charting of voiding and incontinence may by itself lead to significant improvement, and a review of the patient's access to toilet by day and night is always helpful with provision of commode or urine bottle where indicated. Measures aimed at improving mobility, reducing evening fluid intake and stopping or reducing evening sedatives or tranquillizers will also be helpful.

Where detrusor instability exists, it is important to establish a good relationship with the patient by indicating that many cases can be greatly helped by simple retraining. This should start with a regime of regular voiding every one or two hours with a view to increasing the interval to 4 hours.

Drug Therapy

It is wrong to assume that urinary incontinence can be managed by writing a prescription for an 'incontinence drug' and even more wrong if this is supplemented by a supply of incontinence pads—this simply indicates to the patient that the doctor expects the incontinence to continue—so be prepared! The use of drugs remains controversial.

Emepronium bromide is a quaternary ammonium compound which is absorbed to a variable degree from the gut. It certainly causes neurological blockade of the bladder musculature, but several studies suggest that oral administration will only rarely lead to therapeutic levels capable of quelling the unruly detrusor muscle. It has some side-effects—blurring of vision, tachycardia, dry mouth and postural hypotension. A most important danger is buccal or oesophageal ulceration when a tablet is allowed to remain in prolonged contact with the mucosa; hence it should never be used where swallowing is difficult and should invariably be washed down with liberal quantities of fluid. The usual dose is 200 mg at night increasing to 400 mg t.i.d. Propantheline bromide has similar effects and tends to be favoured by urologists in a dose of 15–45 mg daily, but again it has powerful and often unacceptable anticholinergic action. Flavoxate hydrochloride is a tertiary ammonium compound acting on smooth muscle to produce relaxation without significant anticholinergic action. It also possesses a useful papaverine like effect on smooth muscle. This drug may be used alone and, if ineffective, could be added to one of the others noted above since its mode of action is different and in lucky patients there may be a synergistic effect. The usual dose is 300–600 mg daily in three divided doses. Calcium antagonists have been tried (flunarizine, nifedipine and terodiline) as well as prostaglandin-synthetase inhibitors (flurbiprofen). The latter appear to have a significant inhibitory effect on the detrusor but their usefulness has been limited by gastrointestinal irritation. Imipramine is a useful drug in controlling uninhibited detrusor activity and its alpha-adrenergic effect is helpful in improving sphincter tone. It is often effective in doses of only 25–50 mg per day which suggests that it has therapeutic effects not associated with its anticholinergic action.

Drug therapy, if it is going to be effective, should produce results within the space of a few weeks, hence incontinence charts should be kept before and after starting treatment, and if no benefit is seen the drug should be stopped.

Where there is an atonic bladder, cholinergic drugs such as bethanecol may be given subcutaneously. Anticholinesterases such as neostigmine may also be tried. Where bladder neck obstruction has been excluded and catheterization yields residual urine of 150 ml or more, bethanecol may be tried in a dose of 2·5 mg subcutaneously every 6 hours.

Orciprenaline, an alpha-receptor stimulator, may improve the closure of the bladder outlet and it may usefully be given along with emepronium or other detrusor sedative.

Where there is a spastic external sphincter or where detrusor–sphincter dyssynergy exists, alpha blockers such as phentolamine or phenoxybenzamine may help. The diagnosis of such dysfunctions, however, is dependent upon complex urodynamic studies and these drugs are capable of producing severe hypotension.

If atrophic vaginitis is diagnosed, oestrogen therapy should be prescribed. This may be achieved by giving ethinyloestradiol 0·01 mg daily or oestrogen cream topically on alternate nights. Replacement therapy must be continued for at least 6 weeks before benefit is to be expected.

Surgery may be indicated for bladder-neck obstruction as in prostatism and pessaries are indicated for significant degrees of prolapse.

The value of pelvic floor exercises and of the use of faradic stimulation is not established. Biofeedback treatment using a vaginal pressure recorder may be helpful in some younger patients but, unfortunately, this treatment requires mental alertness which is often diminished in older women with detrusor instability associated with dementia.

Aids for Incontinent Patients

Pads and pants may be helpful, especially in females with stress incontinence or minor degrees of urge incontinence. The popular Kanga pants are bulky and often unwelcome to patients. They also require more manual dexterity than some old patients possess. 'Maxi plus' pants are elastic, more easily managed and less bulky.

For men, various devices exist such as the condom urinal or Paul's tubing attached to a urine bag. Often these cannot be firmly attached in obese patients or where there is hernia or hydrocoele.

The numerous devices marketed for women have been singularly unsuccessful. Urine bottles are useful for some men at night, but clumsiness may lead to spillage so that the net result is no benefit. Urine bottles with a 'spill proof' one-way valve in the neck may overcome this problem.

Catheterization is usually to be regarded as a last resort and never should be employed as a long-term measure until an accurate assessment has been made. Infection is generally inevitable and crystal formation in the lumen may lead to blockage and urinary bypass. Over 1–2 years, infection associated with a catheter is usually benign, but beyond this period ascending infection and pyelonephritis become more likely. 'Catheter fever' is common especially after a change of catheter and very serious Gram-negative septicaemia may supervene at any stage. This occurrence may be minimized by a 3-day course of antibiotics over the period of catheter change. Urinary antiseptics may reduce bacterial overgrowth and hence limit crystal formation. Hexamine releases formaldehyde in the urine and is effective against *Escherichia coli* but not against *Proteus*. Nalidixic acid inhibits bacterial DNA synthesis and is effective against *E. coli*, *Proteus* and *Klebsiella* but not *Pseudomonas*. This drug may cause marrow depression and allergic reactions.

Infection in a catheterized patient is not an indication for treatment unless it is symptomatic; all that happens is that a relatively 'innocent' bacterium will be replaced by a much more 'troublesome' one.

Catheter blockage is usually due to deposition of protein and calcium or phosphate salts which some patients seem especially prone to produce. Various bladder washout regimes have been proposed to minimize this; some believe that simple tap water is as good as any. Various types of catheter are available from the simple rubber Foley to the silicone-coated variety. The latter is more expensive but lasts up to 3 months compared to 2–3 weeks for the rubber variety. Short catheters are available for female patients. A 14–16 FG catheter with 5 ml of saline in the bulb should be tried first and often will be successful. Larger amounts of liquid in the bulb may stimulate the detrusor and cause leakage of urine or even extrusion of the catheter. Emepronium (or other drugs mentioned above) may reduce unwelcome detrusor activity and consequent leakage. Good fluid intake should be ensured and regular effective bowel habit. Catheter bags should be hidden for the preservation of the patients' dignity. The bag should be readily and securely fastened to the catheter, easy to empty and in an unobstrusive site. For men the bag should be strapped to the outer calf, and in women either a thigh or a waist bag used (Shepheard sporran). A larger night bag is useful and may encourage restful slumber. Most important, is that patient and/or carer know how to summon expert help should a catheter cause problems, and a sterile pack and spare catheter should always be left in the patient's home for emergency use by general practitioner or nurse.

Other useful aids are plastic drawsheets which are, however, non-absorbable, uncomfortable and unsuitable for long-term use and may predispose to pressure sores. Incontinence pads are useful for short-term use in transient incontinence, but in established cases they present considerable disposal problems. The Kylie sheet can absorb about 1 litre of urine through a hydrophobic membrane which keeps the patient dry. This is a useful device costing about £20 and is suitable for washing in a machine.

Illustrative Case

Mrs B. McC., aged 84, lived alone on the ground floor of a large, unheated house. She suffered from osteoarthritis of her knees and had sustained a fractured neck of the femur in the past. She had been troubled by urinary frequency and urge and stress incontinence since the birth of a daughter 55 years earlier. A pelvic floor repair had not helped very much.

For a year or two before admission to the geriatric service she had struggled with deteriorating mobility and increasing urinary incontinence. She coped by using large numbers of sanitary towels and managed to conceal her problem well. One night in winter she fell in the bathroom and was admitted to the geriatric assessment ward with hypothermia. This catastrophe unmasked her urinary difficulty, of which she was very ashamed.

A continence chart showed that she needed to pass urine every 30 minutes during the day and night, with several episodes of nocturnal incontinence. An MSU grew *E. coli* 10^6/ml, and a 10-day course of ampicillin reduced the urinary frequency a little. Vaginal examination revealed a moderate cystocoele and senile vaginitis, which was treated with local oestrogen cream. Physiotherapy and adequate analgesia improved her mobility, and the provision of a bedside commode reduced the episodes of nocturnal incontinence. The prescription of a small dose of imipramine (25 mg) at night in place of her usual benzodiazepine hypnotic further helped the nocturia. The occupational therapist helped Mrs B. McC. to move into one well-heated room at home, with commode and chemical toilet.

She was an anxious woman (this had contributed to her urinary frequency on admission) and was much reassured by the prescription of pants and absorbable pads, which she wore day and night, although she was rarely wet.

This case illustrates the multifactorial nature of many cases of urinary incontinence, and the way in which a miserable condition may be concealed for a long time. This lady did not undergo urodynamic studies: these can be very useful, but are not universally available and often an empirical approach is successful.

Continence Nursing Adviser

Many district health authorities now employ nurses who are experts in providing advice for incontinent patients. Their function is education and the provision of appropriate appliances. They establish good relationships with patients and carers, ensuring adequate hydration, regular bowel movements, etc. They also help patients and relatives to keep accurate charts and records and advise on drug therapy. They complement rather than usurp the function of the usual community nurses.

Laundry Service

In some areas the provision of a laundry service for patients with urinary incontinence helps sufferers and carers to cope in their own homes.

SUMMARY AND CONCLUSION

A very large majority of patients with urinary incontinence can be greatly relieved and many rendered fully continent by careful management. The programme of treatment for each patient must be based upon careful history taking and examination. Most cases are capable of being satisfactorily managed by a general practitioner and his nursing colleagues. More complex cases should be referred for expert assessment at the earliest stage before morale of patient and carers has suffered serious setback.

The algorithm (*Fig.* 5.2) is based upon that of Hilton and Stanton (1981) and may help practitioners to develop a rational approach to the elucidation of the cause of incontinence and also indicate when referral should be made to a specialist.

This is a field in which general practitioners should become expert since the ageing of the population will certainly lead to many more patients with incontinence in the future. Otherwise Isaacs' (1981) lament will become only too true: 'The greatest tragedy is to issue repeat prescripions for an ineffective drug to a miserable patient whose incontinence could be diagnosed by a finger in the rectum and cured by a resectoscope in the urethra.'

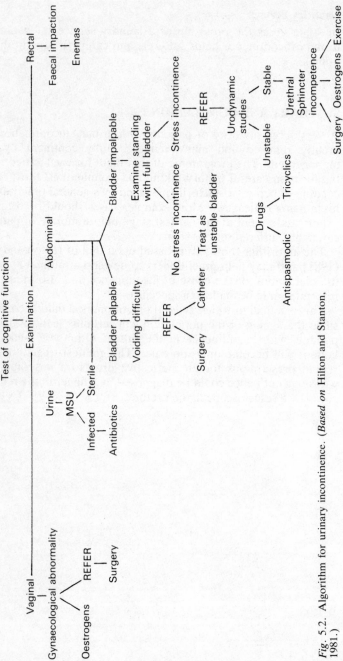

Fig. 5.2. Algorithm for urinary incontinence. (*Based on* Hilton and Stanton, 1981.)

FAECAL INCONTINENCE

The large bowel has two functions:
  a. To extract water from bowel contents
  b. To store faecal material prior to defaecation

The circular muscle of the colon performs a mixing and churning function which encourages bacterial degradation of contents and facilitates water absorption. The longitudinal muscle provides for the onward propulsion of contents by peristalsis. Two or three mass movements occur per day in relation to the gastrocolic reflex.

Faecal continence is maintained by the coordination of visceral and somatic muscle action. The visceral part consists of the smooth muscle of the circular and longitudinal layers of the colon. These muscles also form the internal anal sphincter which is under autonomic control involving sacral cord segments 2–4. The somatic component comprises the muscles of the pelvic floor: external sphincter, puborectalis and iliococcygeus which together form the levator ani (*Fig.* 5.3).

While the external sphincter is under reflex control it can be tightened by conscious effort, but this can be sustained for only a limited period of time, usually about 1 minute. The skeletal muscles have a double function—to prevent herniation of the rectum and lower bowel and to preserve continence. The levator ani fans out to prevent herniation while the puborectalis forms a sling to maintain the sharp angulation of the rectum. This acts as a flap valve mechanism to prevent faeces from descending inappropriately into the lower rectum (*Fig.* 5.4). The internal sphincter is in tonic contraction.

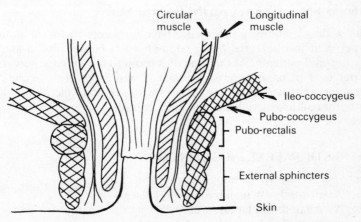

Fig. 5.3. Scheme of muscles at anorectal region.

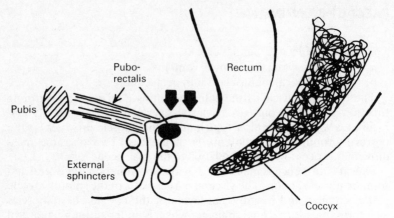

Fig. 5.4. Anorectal junction showing flap valve and puborectalis muscle.

When the lower colon becomes full of faeces and especially in response to the gastrocolic reflex, a bolus of faeces enters the rectum and the resultant distension causes stimulation of stretch receptors, which are believed to lie in the levator ani muscles rather than in the rectal wall itself. This activates a reflex arc (segments 2–4) similar to the micturition reflex. If circumstances permit, the subject adopts a sitting, squatting posture, exerts sufficient abdominal pressure, the internal sphincter relaxes and the puborectalis no longer maintains the flap valve angulation of the rectum thus allowing defaecation to take place.

PREVALENCE OF FAECAL INCONTINENCE

Very wide variations in prevalence have been reported from about 12 per cent in residential home populations to 66 per cent in long-stay hospital patients. At the time of referral to our geriatric service, 10 per cent of patients have 'occasional' and 2 per cent 'frequent' faecal incontinence. In nearly all cases with persistent faecal incontinence there is associated loss of bladder control.

CAUSES OF FAECAL INCONTINENCE

There are three main aetiological groups:
- *a*. Associated with underlying bowel disease
- *b*. Associated with faecal stasis
- *c*. Associated with neurological disorders

a. Cases with Underlying Bowel Disease

Many common diseases may be accompanied by faecal incontinence—carcinoma of rectum or lower colon, diverticular disease and rectal prolapse. Less common are ischaemic colitis, proctitis, ulcerative colitis, Crohn's disease and megacolon. Diarrhoeal conditions may lead to incontinence as in diabetic autonomic neuropathy, acute infections and occasionally in malabsorption. Excessive use of laxatives may cause incontinence as may iron salts, mefenamic acid and many antibiotics.

b. Cases Associated with Bowel Stasis

This is by far the commonest cause of faecal incontinence in geriatric practice. Its detection is very important since it can almost always be controlled, although this may be difficult and take considerable time to achieve.

Transit time in old age is prolonged even in healthy subjects and it may be 72 hours or longer compared to 24–48 hours in younger individuals. Hence constipation may readily supervene, especially when mobility is impaired and dietary fibre and fluid intake are inadequate. Common precipitating factors are acute illness such as infection or injury, especially when hospital admission occurs.

Two main types of constipation are described. The first is the 'colonic' type in which transit is greatly slowed, more water being absorbed leaving hard and rather dry faeces which are often difficult to pass and may cause painful defaecation. The other is the 'dyschezic' type in which transit time may be normal or only slightly prolonged, but for unknown reasons the contents are delayed in their passage from descending colon into sigmoid colon and rectum. This eventually results in a large putty-like mass in the terminal colon and rectum which is very difficult to expel.

Both varieties may lead to faecal impaction, in one with hard 'cannon balls' and in the other with putty-like material which may leak and cause smearing of clothes and bedding. There may also be outpouring of mucus from rectal glands which presents as spurious bypass diarrhoea. The two types can usually be differentiated by rectal examination and the extent of colonic stasis may be revealed by a plain abdominal radiograph. When the rectum remains distended for prolonged periods, the sphincters lose tone and the anus becomes patulous with incontinence. In almost all cases of severe stasis the rectum is affected and so the diagnosis can be made by rectal examination.

Illustrative Case

Mrs J. G. was an 81-year-old widow who had been resident in a local authority old people's home for 3 years. She remained very independent until the arthritis of her knees started to affect her mobility and she was started on dihydrocodeine, 2 tablets t.i.d. Over the next month her mobility failed to improve and the staff noticed first episodes of urinary incontinence and more recently diarrhoea with faecal incontinence. Her general practitioner was called and, on examination, found a mass in her left iliac fossa. On examining her rectum, he found a large, hard faecal mass which had stretched the external sphincter to a degree where the anal canal was incompetent. A manual evacuation was required initially, followed by a series of small bulk phosphate enemas given by the district nurse which gradually emptied the rectum. The dihydrocodeine was replaced by piroxicam and she was referred to the geriatric service for physiotherapy at the day hospital. Both her urinary and faecal incontinence resolved as her lower bowel was cleared and a normal bowel habit re-established with a high-fibre diet and occasional oral aperient.

Recent studies have shown that two types of rectal dysfunction exist, one in which there appears to be marked reduction in sensitivity so that the patient is barely aware of a distended balloon in the rectum, while in the other type the rectum appears hypersensitive and will expel the balloon after only slight distension. It is tempting to regard the first example as analogous to the atonic neurogenic bladder (*see above*), while the second resembles the uninhibited neurogenic bladder.

c. Cases Associated with Neurological Disorders

The neurological disorders may be either local or central. Recent research has shown neuronal degeneration with myopathic changes in large bowel biopsies from old subjects, and it is conjectured that these changes may be associated with prolonged and repeated stretching of nerves from frequent straining at stool. This suggests that a vicious circle may be established with 'primary' constipation leading to prolonged straining which, in turn, leads to neuronal damage and worsening constipation.

Degeneration of the myenteric plexus is well documented as a result of laxative abuse and may also result from excessive use of anticholinergic drugs or phenothiazines. This may lead to sphincter laxity, diminished sensitivity of the anal canal and decreased tone in the puborectalis muscle, which interferes with the important flap-valve mechanism associated with rectal angulation as described above.

Although these local defects are important in individual patients, central lesions are much more common. Thus central inhibitory control may be diminished as in the uninhibited neurogenic bladder.

This is usually associated with dementia in which formed stools are passed once or twice daily in response to rectal distension without the over-riding effect of cortical inhibition. In these cases formed stools will be passed into clothes or bedding often in association with a gastrocolic reflex. This type of incontinence is readily distinguished from the faecal smearing and spurious diarrhoea described above.

MANAGEMENT AND TREATMENT

Where a remediable condition is responsible for the incontinence this should be diagnosed and treated. A review should be held of all medications (prescribed and 'across the counter') and a careful history obtained. Clinical assessment must include mental testing and rectal examination.

Most cases of impaction will be revealed by putting a finger in the rectum.

Where there is diverticular disease, a high-fibre diet should be prescribed with or without a bulking agent such as ispaghula. Any drug liable to cause diarrhoea or constipation should be withdrawn.

Faecal stasis should be treated initially by seeking to clear the terminal gut with phosphate enemas (or simple soap and water) or suppositories of bisacodyl. Once the terminal 'plug' has been removed, then a regular laxative regime should be instituted usually with an irritant type of drug such as bisacodyl. Where stasis is severe and has been prolonged, the re-establishment of regular bowel habit may take weeks or even months and may necessitate such distressing manoeuvres as manual disimpaction, oral mannitol or even whole gut irrigation which, of course, require specialist assistance. It is essential that cases should be detected early and patient distress thus minimized and hospital admission avoided if possible.

Once the lower bowel has been cleared and some sort of regular habit achieved, it is important to prevent recurrence. This necessitates encouragement towards fuller mobility, adequate dietary fibre (30 g per day) and a regular fluid intake of 1·5–2·0 litres per day.

Where central neurological damage is an important causative factor with precipitate evacuation of formed stools, the plan should be to induce constipation by sedating the hyperactive reflexes by means of codeine phosphate 15–30 mg t.i.d. Thereafter evacuation may be achieved in a purposive fashion by giving enemas two or three times per week, usually after a meal when the gastrocolic reflex may thus be augmented.

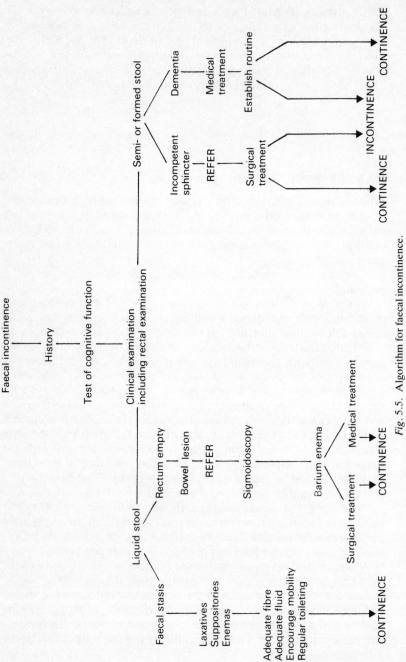

Fig. 5.5. Algorithm for faecal incontinence.

SUMMARY AND CONCLUSION

Faecal incontinence is common, very distressing and usually preventable. It leads to severe demoralization of patients and readily causes carers to despair and to give up the struggle hence leading to institutional care. Careful history taking and simple clinical examination will reveal the underlying cause in a large majority of cases and effective control is usually possible by simple treatment based upon an understanding of pathophysiology.

The accompanying algorithm (*Fig.* 5.5) may help practitioners to adopt a systematic approach to this problem.

REFERENCES

Hilton P. and Stanton S. L. (1981) Algorithmic method for assessing urinary incontinence in elderly women. *Br. Med. J.* **282**, 940.
Isaacs B. (1981) Incontinence in the elderly. *Prescribers' J.* **2**, 285.

SUGGESTED READING

Brocklehurst J. C. (ed.) (1984) *Urology in the Elderly.* Edinburgh: Churchill Livingstone.
Mandelstam D. (ed.) (1980) *Incontinence and its Management.* Beckenham: Croom Helm.

6 STROKE AND TRANSIENT ISCHAEMIC ATTACKS

For patients and their families stroke often spells disaster. The colloquial Scottish term for stroke is 'shock' which conveys the impression of suddenness and calamity more forcibly.

It is probably impossible for the non-sufferer to imagine the despair and hopelessness which overcome the individual when, in the space of a few minutes or hours, he is transformed from a healthy, independent and intelligent person into a helpless, immobile, incontinent patient, sometimes unable to speak or even to swallow.

Strokes are now the third commonest cause of death (after ischaemic heart disease and cancer). Approximately one-third of stroke patients die within the first 3 weeks, another third regain independent living, while the remaining third survive but in a state of varying dependency. The burden of stroke upon the health and social services is immense. Garraway (1976) has pointed out that in Scotland in 1973, 11·2 per cent of hospital bed days were used by stroke patients (excluding only mental illness and subnormality beds), representing substantially more than 1 million bed days (in a country with 5 million inhabitants). The proportion of bed days for stroke patients rises with age, being over 20 per cent for females aged 75 or more (Garraway, 1976).

We shall use Marshall's definition of stroke as 'a persisting neurological deficit due to a cerebrovascular lesion' (Marshall, 1979). Strokes are divided into cerebral infarctions and haemorrhages. The former are associated with obstruction of a cerebral artery due to thrombosis or embolism, while the latter are due to rupture of a cerebral vessel leading to intracerebral or subarachnoid haemorrhage. Cerebral haemorrhage is now much less commonly diagnosed than previously, presumably mainly due to more accurate diagnosis. Three-quarters of strokes are due to infarction and within this group it is now known that about 45 per cent are associated with embolus. The common sources of cerebral embolus are the heart in atrial fibrillation (especially in the presence of rheumatic mitral stenosis), detached mural thrombus in acute myocardial infarction and atheromatous plaques in the internal carotid arteries or associated with stenosis of such arteries. Predisposing factors are hypertension, diabetes mellitus and conditions associated with high haematocrit levels (polycythaemia rubra vera or secondary polycythaemia), which lead to marked increase in blood viscosity and corresponding reduction in cerebral perfusion.

Intracranial space-occupying lesions may mimic stroke, but in most cases a careful history will provide suggestive evidence especially if the onset has been of slow evolution as opposed to the abruptness of stroke.

EPIDEMIOLOGY

It is believed that there are about 130 000 persons in the UK who suffer from some stroke-related disability.

Incidence and prevalence increase steeply with age:

Age group	New strokes per 1000 persons per year
55–64	3
65–74	8
75+	25

This means that a practice which has a disproportionately larger number of very old patients will have many more stroke patients than the average.

Garraway (1976) has used figures from the Office of Population Censuses and Surveys to calculate the burden of stroke upon an average Scottish practice (2010 persons) in one year.

The total number of consultations with stroke patients was 76, 54 of whom were visited at home. Of the 24 requiring referral, 10 were referred to hospital for admission, 5 to hospital as outpatients, 3 for laboratory investigation, 2 for community services and 4 for other agencies.

Of the 23 separate episodes of stroke, 12 were new, 9 required follow-up care, 1 was a recurrence and there was 1 episode which did not come directly to the general practitioner's notice and was admitted as an emergency direct to hospital.

In the past four decades there has been a remarkable decline in the incidence of strokes, especially in the USA. Work from the Mayo Clinic, for example, has shown that for every 100 strokes in the population of Rochester, Minnesota, in 1945–9, there were only 55 in 1970 and the decline persists. It is tempting to attribute this great improvement to earlier, more widespread and more effective control of hypertension plus greater health consciousness (reduction of fat in diet, emphasis upon regular exercise, etc.), but many epidemiologists remain sceptical about this relationship since the downward trend was apparent before these preventive factors were substantially in operation.

Many now regard isolated atrial fibrillation as an important risk factor for stroke. Thus Kannel *et al.* (1978) found that subjects with atrial fibrillation had six times the incidence of stroke compared to the rest of the population. A patient with atrial fibrillation who has had a stroke is at high risk of a further stroke in the ensuing few months.

PATHOPHYSIOLOGY OF STROKE

Haemorrhagic strokes are believed to be mainly due to the rupture of perforating arteries in hypertensive subjects. The leaked blood may form an intracerebral haematoma but there is blood in the cerebrospinal fluid in 80 per cent of cases.

Infarctions are much more complex and the supplying artery, although the site of atheromatous change, may not be blocked. The underlying cause is then an alteration in the haemodynamics of cerebral perfusion as may occur when there is occlusion of one or more of the four main extracerebral arteries of the neck which supply blood to the circle of Willis. Similarly cerebral infarction may result when there is a sudden drop in blood pressure or cardiac output, as in acute myocardial infarction or a large intestinal haemorrhage.

CLINICAL FEATURES

The picture in stroke is infinitely variable and no two strokes are ever identical, with the picture being influenced by the site of the lesion, its extent and the speed with which it develops.

The middle cerebral artery territory is most frequently involved, right and left hemispheres being equally often affected.

The following functions may show disturbance.

Motor Function

Initially there is flaccid paralysis on the affected side which usually gradually gives way to a state of increased tone. If this is allowed to continue, it may lead to severe spasticity and uncontrollable clonus which can both be severely disabling and lead to painful spasms and later to flexion contractures.

Motor loss is usually more marked in the arm, but where the anterior cerebral artery is affected, this picture may be reversed.

Motor loss, although important, is rarely so significant as other losses noted below in determining success or failure in rehabilitation.

Sensory Function

Pain and touch sensation may be absent on the affected side and this is easily detected by standard neurological examination.

Proprioceptive loss is common and its detection is essential for the evolution of a suitable rehabilitation programme. Proprioception is most appropriately tested by the thumb-finding test (Allison, 1966). The patient is asked to grasp the thumb of the affected hand with the good hand and eyes open. This should be done a few times to familiarize the patient, then the patient's eyes are covered, the affected hand moved and the patient told to grasp the affected thumb. Slight loss will cause the patient to be rather uncertain of the affected hand's position, but it is secured without too much fumbling. Severe loss means that the patient has no idea where the affected limb is in space. He may eventually identify the affected forearm and then climb this to get to the hand and finally the thumb.

Much more subtle sensory disturbances may occur when the parietal region is affected, especially in the non-dominant hemisphere. In these cases the patient may show little awareness of his left arm and leg and may even neglect them totally. Sometimes he may deny that the limbs belong to him and may even claim that they belong to someone nearby. It is a good rule always to inspect stroke patients from a distance in a covert fashion before approaching them. The patient with significant neglect of the left side will be seen to sit slumped to the left, with the left arm dangling pointlessly over the side of the bed or chair, while the patient seems to be peering into a world which only exists on his right side. Our practice with stroke patients (especially with left hemiplegia) is always to approach them and stand on the affected side, preferably placing someone else on the good side. When the examiner speaks to the patient it may be observed that the patient replies to the person on their good side, strongly suggestive of neglect. Confirmation of this finding can be obtained from asking the patient to fill in the figures on an empty clock face or to pick up matchsticks scattered widely over a board placed before the patient. In either case the patient appears to pay little or no attention to objects on the left half. The occupational therapist will quickly spot this deficit in patients who claim to be fully dressed, despite the fact that they have made no attempt to put their left arm into its sleeve.

Obviously this dysfunction, especially if severe, makes successful rehabilitation less likely, especially if accompanied by personality change and incontinence. These patients often become very demanding and unrealistic, while their constant denial that they are at all disabled is very destructive of morale among their carers.

The full-blown syndrome of neglect is rare in persons with right hemiparesis, but minor disturbances of perception are more common than previously believed to be the case.

Visual Disturbances

Where the stroke affects the optic radiations, homonymous hemianopia will occur on the side of the affected limbs. While this is a serious deficit, it is not so likely to interfere with rehabilitation as do neglect syndromes because once the patient realizes that he has defective vision on one side he can scan to that side by rotating his head, thus compensating to some extent for the hemianopia.

Disturbances of Speech

Dysphasia

About two-thirds of patients with right hemiplegia will have some speech disturbance associated with damage to the speech centres, which are mainly in the temporoparietal lobes of the dominant hemisphere.

Speech is an extremely complex function and the mechanisms involved are incompletely understood. In very general terms, however, there are two main types of dysphasia. One is expressive dysphasia in which the patient has difficulty in finding words but appears to understand all or most of what is said (or written). Receptive dysphasia occurs in patients who have diminished (or absent) comprehension of spoken or written words and who may talk in a largely meaningless, disconnected and jargon fashion. Pure examples of expressive or receptive dysphasia are rare and most with expressive problems will show some comprehension deficit which may be more marked at some times than others, e.g. when the patient is tired or distressed.

Patients with marked dysphasia suffer severe emotional stress and often become very frustrated with outbursts of anger and sometimes aggression. Hence the strain upon their families may also be severe and they deserve special support and help.

In strokes affecting the vertebrobasilar territory there may be dysarthria in which slurred indistinct speech occurs due to incoordination and imbalance of the neuromuscular control of speech.

This is often a temporary disability, except in those cases with progressive cerebrovascular disease in whom the picture merges into that of pseudobulbar palsy with limb weakness and spasticity, dysphagia and emotional lability.

Apraxia

This condition implies the loss of ability to perform learned actions in the absence of significant motor or sensory loss. In the upper limb it may result in the patient simply not using the arm despite good muscle power and the ability to flex and extend the joints. The arm is then 'carried about like a parcel by the patient' (in the words of one of our physiotherapy colleagues). Lesions of the dominant parietal lobe may produce bilateral deficits which may affect the movements of lips and tongue or cause inability to walk. Such a patient when laid on a couch can move his legs normally on command, yet when asked to walk his legs simply cannot initiate and sustain the purposive movements of walking.

Mental Disturbances

Mental Confusion

Some degree of mental confusion occurs in many stroke patients in the immediate aftermath of the acute episode. Relatives and doctors then wait anxiously to see whether this is only a manifestation of the acute cerebral dysfunction brought on by the vascular event or whether it portends longer-lasting and irreversible cerebral damage. When confusion persists, this is a most unfavourable prognostic sign for recovery of useful function.

Sometimes the initial confusion clears completely, but the patient thereafter shows limited ability to cope with abstract ideas and hence with new learning or understanding. Patients also frequently have a poor attention span and are easily distracted, which again makes rehabilitation more difficult and independence less likely.

It is important to realize that a patient with significant perceptual disturbance and unilateral neglect may appear confused, but is in reality trying to come to terms with his new world which has been cleft in two and large chunks of one-half cast away.

Depression

The catastrophe of stroke is so overwhelming that dejection and despair are to be expected and team members must do everything to encourage the patient and indicate improvement as it occurs (however meagre it may be).

True depression is, however, also common and may occur at any stage in the first few months. Its advent must be carefully sought since there is no hope of successful rehabilitation in untreated depressed stroke patients. Where the patient retains normal ability to communicate, suitable inquiry may be made along the lines outlined in the appendix to Chapter 8 (p. 156). Much greater problems arise, however, in aphasic or dysphasic patients who cannot accurately express their feelings and may have decreased comprehension. In these circumstances all team members should watch carefully for telltale signs: a depressed look with a fixed frown, any evidence of diurnal variation with the patient being worse in the morning, poor appetite and insomnia. Patients may appear withdrawn and indicate widespread pain and discomfort (including headache) without obvious physical basis. In these cases, a trial of an antidepressant is mandatory.

Incontinence

After a stroke urinary incontinence is usually associated with diminished cortical inhibition of the spontaneous contractions of the bladder detrusor (*see* Chapter 5).

In the acute stage urinary retention may occur with overflow and regular palpation of the lower abdomen should be done daily at this stage.

Stroke patients are prone to constipation which may, if unheeded, proceed to faecal impaction of the rectum with overflow incontinence. This is a common source of discomfort and embarrassment to patients and a considerable stress to carers for whom it may be 'the last straw'. Bowel movements should be regularly charted and a rectal examination done every 2 days until the rehabilitation is well under way and the patient is eating and drinking normally and beginning to mobilize.

Epilepsy

Occasionally a stroke will produce epileptic fits in the acute phase but more commonly epilepsy occurs later on. About 1 in 20 stroke patients will eventually require anticonvulsant therapy. The temporary paresis which occasionally follows a fit (Todd's paralysis) should be recognized as a post-ictal phenomenon and the patient should not be labelled as a stroke (or TIA—transient ischaemic attack) victim.

PROGNOSIS IN STROKE

Prognosis as regards survival depends on the nature of the stroke, its site and size. Haemorrhagic strokes have a higher death rate with 75 per cent dead at 6 months compared to under half of cerebral infarction cases. Embolic cases fare worse than those with thrombotic strokes.

The initial level of consciousness is a good prognostic guide (Oxbury *et al.* 1975).

Level of consciousness	Percentage dead at 3 weeks
Fully conscious	Nil
Drowsy/confused	30
Unresponsive	50

Patients in older age groups have a poorer prognosis and those with total leg and arm paralysis have an early mortality, thrice that of those who retain some limb movement.

The prognosis for successful rehabilitation to some level of independent existence is much more complex and uncertain, being dependent upon many factors, some of which are very difficult to quantify. Factors which carry a poor prognosis are:

1. *Poor motivation.* Nurses and therapists will soon form an opinion on patients' determination to overcome their disability. Phrases such as 'She seems unwilling to try' or 'He would just sit and let others do everything for him' are ominous. The general practitioner's and community nurses' advice may be invaluable here since they are often able to shed light on the patient's previous personality. Was this always a passive person or was he or she a hardworking individual? If reports of low motivation after a stroke conflict with previous evidence of determination and rugged independence, then a cause should be sought and depression seriously considered.

Illustrative Case

Mr H. M., a 70-year-old retired, right-handed carpenter, was referred in March 1985, having been discharged 2 days earlier from a medical ward where he had spent 3 weeks. The discharge report said that he had suffered a stroke, had aphasia and 'multi-infarct dementia'.

He had lived contentedly with his 67-year-old wife in a ground-floor flat. His wife had been found to have breast cancer a year earlier and was receiving tamoxifen. She seemed fit and vigorous and was very anxious to support her husband at home.

His right arm showed moderate weakness and clumsiness, but there was no proprioceptive loss. His right leg was only slightly affected and he could walk with encouragement. He had marked dysphasia with almost no word power. It was uncertain how much he could understand.

Day-hospital attendance was arranged and there further detailed assessment was commenced. He could walk but seemed rather unwilling to make the effort and he needed much prompting and cajoling to wash and dress himself. After 2 weeks it became obvious that he was worse, having falls and nocturnal incontinence. His wife also reported that she was having great difficulty in getting him to eat and drink. He was therefore admitted to the geriatric ward where he was found to be slightly dehydrated.

Neurological signs were unchanged, but now he could only walk with much help and could no longer wash or dress himself and was frequently incontinent.

His degree of dependency seemed much worse than would be expected from his neurological state and causes other than stroke were considered. The first possibility seemed to be a space-occupying intracranial lesion, but CT scan showed only evidence of a left parietal infarct.

Reports now came in from geriatric team members which suggested another possible diagnosis. The nurses said that he seemed very withdrawn and quite often would turn away from anyone who approached him and tried to communicate (including his, by now, very distressed wife). Nurses also described how he would from time to time clutch his epigastrium and evince signs of severe distress. We attempted a barium meal at this stage but he could not cooperate. Physiotherapists and occupational therapists also reported that he seemed generally very unhappy and withdrawn and would only eat and drink after much coaxing.

A diagnosis of depression was made and he started to take imipramine. With 50 mg of this drug he developed quite severe postural hypotension so mianserin was substituted. Within 2–3 weeks he was a changed individual— cooperating well in his rehabilitation, continent and now appearing to understand a good deal of what was said to him. He was eating well and regaining lost weight. He was discharged after 8 weeks to attend the day hospital. Close contact was kept with his wife through the health visitor attached to his general practitioner. A continuing problem was that his wife had to help him with micturition twice a night and she found this interruption rather tiring. She was advised to have a holiday with her daughter in West Scotland in October 1985 and arrangements were made for him to be looked after in a residential home. In April 1986 his wife suffered a recurrence of breast cancer with skeletal metastasis, and the geriatric service, oncologists and primary care team are collaborating to ensure that husband and wife have the care and treatment that they now need.

This case illustrates the importance of remembering that failure in stroke rehabilitation may be associated with depression. It also underlines the importance of team assessment in diagnosis and of close collaboration between the geriatric service, the general practitioner and other specialists involved in the spouse's medical care.

2. *Persistent incontinence* has a poor prognosis for useful recovery.

3. *Severe perceptual disturbances*, if persistent, diminish the chance of successful rehabilitation.

Illustrative Case

Mr W. F., a retired postman, lived in a third-floor flat with his fit 64-year-old wife. Two sons lived nearby and there was a moderate amount of contact. Mr W. F. was an extremely fit man until aged 67 when he had a stroke on Christmas Eve. He suddenly felt numbness in his left arm and his wife noted that his mouth was 'twisted'. Over the space of a few hours he had marked loss of power in his left arm, some weakness of the left leg and an obvious left facial weakness. His wife said that 'He never understood that he had had a stroke'. He was admitted to a general medical unit (his practitioner admitted afterwards that he would have referred Mr W. F. to the geriatric service but believed that he was 'well under 65'). There he appeared to be stable and over the next few days the left-sided weakness decreased a little. Because there was a severe influenza epidemic medical beds were desperately needed and he was sent home with an arrangement to be admitted shortly for rehabilitation in another hospital. This led to severe stress on his wife who was struggling to cope with her husband's immobility, frequent incontinence and increasing irascibility. After 3 weeks he was admitted to another hospital but he did not fare well at all. Both he and his wife claim that they were told he would never walk again. Mr W. F. said that he just sat in a wheelchair all day apart from 15 minutes in the physiotherapy department. He was discharged home after 3 weeks with a recommendation that he should be referred to the geriatric service.

At the initial home visit he was found to be cognitively intact but had moderate neglect of his left side and still did not appreciate that he had had a stroke. There was some proprioceptive loss on the left side but testing for this was complicated by the neglect. He also had a painful and stiff left shoulder which interfered with sleep, making it difficult for him to get into a comfortable position. He was angry and bitter and tended to vent his frustration upon his wife—even to the extent of blaming her for the stroke.

He attended the day hospital where the team agreed that there were several priorities:

1. To help him to achieve awareness of his left side. This was done by constant exhortation and by making him walk in parallel bars in front of a mirror. He was discouraged from using his right arm as a substitute for the left.
2. To treat the painful shoulder by non-steroidal anti-inflammatory medication and local heat.
3. To get him walking as soon as possible as the best means of restoring his and his wife's morale. This meant taking some short cuts and in some respects not adhering to strict physiotherapy standards, but all agreed that for a person like Mr W. F. we had to produce tangible results.

He cooperated enthusiastically and made steady progress. A few weeeks later his wife strained her back so he was admitted to the ward for 3 weeks after which he was mobile with a walking stick, his shoulder was much improved and he needed only minor help in getting his left arm into sleeves, etc.

He continued to improve for fully 9 months after which he could manage the three flights of stairs to his flat.

This case illustrates the importance of team assessment and the necessity for a treatment and rehabilitation plan. Above all it emphasizes the importance of the initial approach of the professional to the stroke patient. It is highly unlikely that anyone actually said: 'You will never walk again' to Mr W. F., but the fact remains that both he and his wife received this message and that their morale was all but irreparably shattered by it.

4. *Existence of other disabling conditions* may adversely affect prospects, e.g. ischaemic heart disease with limited exercise tolerance, chronic obstructive airways disease, obesity and severe arthropathy (especially of weightbearing joints).

TREATMENT

The treatment in the acute phase of stroke is to a large extent concerned with maintaining life and preventing complications. The unconscious or drowsy patient must be properly positioned to secure a clear airway and turned 2-hourly to prevent pressure damage to tissues. Where there is urinary retention, catheterization will be needed, but we do not believe that this should be done for incontinence *per se*. Attention must be paid to securing adequate fluid intake (and this may be judged by urinary output where it is possible to measure it). Mouth hygiene should be meticulously attended to and a careful guard mounted against faecal impaction.

In recent years efforts have been directed at specific treatment in the acute phase to reduce the volume of destroyed brain tissue. This has quite a powerful rationale since, although each infarction or haemorrhage will cause death of tissue in its centre, there is a surrounding area (the penumbra) which, although damaged and not functionally normal, may still be receiving some degree of perfusion. Animal experiments have shown that brain tissue can survive several hours of only 50 per cent normal perfusion and yet recover more or less normal function. The nature of the changes in the penumbra is not certain but, on the basis that some of the underperfusion may be due to oedema, controlled trials have been made of treatments to reduce this. Thus i.v. glycerol or mannitol has been used, as has dexamethasone. Sadly, no benefits have been shown and the latter treatment is not without risks so at present such procedures are not recommended. Some workers, however, argue that these trials were defective in design since many patients did not commence their treatment for several hours (as much as 18 hours) after the stroke by which time reversibility is impossible.

Very occasionally, an intracerebral haematoma may have to be surgically evacuated, but this must be very rare in older patients in the UK. The chance of survival in a very damaged and dependent state, after such intervention, is high and many would question its ethical justification especially in older patients.

REHABILITATION

This is probably the most important consideration for primary care workers. The patient needs support, explanation and reassurance to come to terms with the fearful consequences of stroke and this may very appropriately come from a well-known and trusted general practitioner. Likewise the wife who sees her previously vigorously independent husband reduced to a state of infantile helplessness needs all the help and understanding she can get. If the husband survives the acute phase to emerge as a bad-tempered, inconsiderate and demanding tyrant she may well exclaim (as many relatives have done to us): 'This is not the person I married; this is a stranger.' The good general practitioner has a unique responsibility both in the acute phase and during rehabilitation to help patient and family to come to terms with what has happened.

We have been told repeatedly by family members how much they longed for explanation and understanding and how much the general practitioner's visits and support are valued. It would be a good idea for primary care teams to work out plans for regular contact with stroke patients and their families so that they feel that continuing interest is being shown and their sense of isolation thus diminished. These issues came out very strongly in the sessions on stroke which we held with general practitioner trainees, stroke victims and their relatives.

Stroke rehabilitation is a complex affair and where the residual disability is of any seriousness it will require prolonged contact with a multidisciplinary team. The notion that the patient merely requires 'intensive physiotherapy' (a largely meaningless term which in some instances may mean 20 minutes daily in a physiotherapy department with an overworked therapist) plus a calliper and some sort of walking stick is naive in the extreme and indicates total ignorance of patients' and families' rehabilitation needs in stroke.

We therefore strongly advise that stroke patients who seem likely to be left with significant disability should be referred for expert assessment. This is especially so in cases with communication problems or perceptual defects. Where is this expert assessment to be done? Obviously, in the few areas where there is a stroke unit then referral should be thereto, although with very old patients (and those with other complex problems) the geriatric service may be more appropriate. Any geriatric service worth its salt will be interested and competent in stroke rehabilitation since these cases constitute a substantial proportion of the work of such a unit.

The first task of the rehabilitation team is to perform full assessment which means identification of all functional deficiencies as outlined above. This is combined with a search for other diseases and an assessment of motivation and personality. Last, but by no means least, the principal carer is seen and her morale, attitudes, expectations and hopes investigated. How much can she be effectively involved in the rehabilitation process?

In our service we encourage the dismantling of demarcation barriers between the different groups involved in rehabilitation. This has been greatly enhanced by having the rehabilitation area in the middle of the ward with bed areas all around. The patients' main day room is adjacent to the rehabilitation area and the whole is open-planned. Hence nurses, physiotherapists and occupational therapists are perforce brought together where patients are being rehabilitated. All staff have expressed approval of this arrangement and like it much better than the traditional pattern whereby patients are spirited away to the physiotherapy department, then to occupational therapy, while the nurses (who have the greatest potential for effective rehabilitation) remain in the ward largely unaware of what has been happening to their patients.

The Nurses' Contribution

Nurses in hospital are with patients 24 hours per day and they therefore have a great influence upon rehabilitation which must continue round the clock. Community nurses likewise have more frequent, intimate and prolonged contact with patients and families than other team members.

They should be instructed by physiotherapists on correct positioning of the patient: to sit upright with the affected arm carefully supported to minimize spasticity and downward drag upon the shoulder joint, which is readily damaged by incorrect positioning and may become subluxated if patients are lifted bodily by an attendant's arm thrust into the armpit. Poor handling of patients at this stage may lead to prolonged and severe pain and stiffness of the affected shoulder. Joints should be passively put through a full range of movement several times daily from the onset of the stroke.

Generally, lockers and visitors should be sited on the affected side so that the patient's awareness of that side is reinforced. Where serious neglect exists, of course, this may be futile since the patient will remain totally unaware of events on this side.

Meticulous attention should be paid to skin, mouth, bowel and bladder. Incontinence should be charted and a regime of regular toileting instituted. Patients should be placed upon a commode or, better still, taken to the toilet at regular intervals to encourage regular voiding.

Community nurses have a similar role but their main function may be to instruct relatives in the optimum care of the patient, e.g. regular careful passive movement of afflicted limbs.

Physiotherapist

The physiotherapist has a most important dual role: to instruct relatives, nurses, etc. in the proper handling of the patient and to be involved directly with the patient to ensure proper positioning, limitation of spasticity and prevention of deformity. Added to this are measures to improve exercise tolerance, balance and coordination.

Together with other team members and with the cooperation of the patient and family, rehabilitation goals should be set, e.g. sitting upright, standing with assistance, walking with assistance and then in parallel bars. It is important that realistic goals should be set otherwise failure to achieve will result in despondency and low morale; the patient may then feel like 'giving up'.

Several specialized physiotherapy techniques have been devised based to a varying degree upon accepted neurophysiology. The fact that all have equally enthusiastic and convinced proponents indicates that none has clear superiority over the others. The enthusiasm of the physiotherapists is perhaps their most important ingredient. Most of these techniques are concerned with relearning lost mechanisms and much use is made of the 'mat room' where patients can become involved in rolling, crawling, kneeling and standing in a protected environment. Such movements certainly help to prevent or minimize spasticity and reinforcement of unhelpful reflexes.

Various walking aids are employed, such as four- or three-legged sticks for patients with poor balance. Sometimes perfectionist physiotherapists will try to prevent or limit reliance upon such aids in the hope that the patient will eventually be able to walk unaided. We recently saw a hemiplegic lady who had been attending for 'outpatient physiotherapy' for 2 years. She could walk quite well with her tripod stick but had been forbidden to use it. The outcome was that any time she wanted to walk about the house her sister had to help her. The tripod meanwhile rested in the corner of their living room unused!

Callipers and toe-raising orthoses are sometimes useful but are rarely required except in cases of severe persistent foot drop.

A knee brace may sometimes allow earlier ambulation and hence improve proprioception and postural control in the early stages of stroke rehabilitation where the knee joint is apt to give way.

Occupational Therapist

In a good rehabilitation department the occupational therapist and physiotherapist overlap and complement each other to a large extent.

The occupational therapist's function is to assess in detail the patient's disability, especially in the more subtle areas of motivation and perceptual defects.

She is responsible for educating the patient in activities of daily living—washing, dressing, toileting, transferring from bed, chair, bath and toilet, and in household tasks such as cooking, making snacks, etc.

Once again, the occupational therapist must be prepared to spend time with relatives in order to ensure that they know what to do and what must be left to the patient.

Various devices are available to help with dressing and feeding and aids may have to be provided in the patient's home before or soon after return, e.g. bath aids, rails at toilet and bath, monkey pole above bed and bed and chair of a special height. These needs are best assessed at a predischarge home visit by patient and occupational therapist. Often it is helpful to have a relative present and sometimes also the community nurse and/or the home help supervisor. (*See* Chapter 9.)

Speech Therapist

Once again, the speech therapist's main function is to assess the nature of the speech disturbance and then instruct others who are with the patient for much longer periods—nurses for patients in hospital and relatives in all cases.

The recent development in the UK of voluntary stroke clubs run by the Chest, Heart and Stroke Association has proved a great success. Patients and their relatives can visit regularly, meet other patients and relatives and learn from each other how to cope with stroke disability. For patients with dysphasia, selected volunteers have proved extremely helpful through meetings in stroke clubs and visiting at home (Eaton-Griffith and Miller, 1980).

Social Worker

The value of the social worker is emphasized in Chapter 9. We have found that a good social worker is often invaluable in helping families to come to terms with the new situation which exists when a member is a stroke victim. She can also ensure that the family receives attendance allowances, mobility allowances, etc. to which they may be entitled.

TRANSIENT ISCHAEMIC ATTACKS

A transient ischaemic attack (TIA) is defined as a focal disturbance of neurological function lasting less than 24 hours ascribable to cerebrovascular disease. Most TIAs last very much less than 24 hours, often only a few minutes to an hour. Some have used the term reversible ischaemic neurological deficit (RIND) for deficits which last more than 24 hours but clear completely within 3 weeks. It seems likely, however, that many of these are really just small strokes.

Pathophysiology

The occurrence of a TIA indicates the existence of a cerebrovascular abnormality which may be a small embolus from a stenosed internal carotid artery or a plaque of atheroma therein. Another cause is an abnormality of an intracerebral artery, such as atherosclerotic narrowing which does not interfere with perfusion unless there is an associated general circulatory deficiency as in states accompanied by a sudden drop in blood pressure (vasovagal attacks, postural hypotension) or cardiac output (paroxysmal cardiac arrhythmia). Hypertension may also lead to TIAs in which case the danger of stroke is very considerable. Cervical spondylosis may lead to vertebrobasilar TIAs as when an osteophyte compresses and occludes a vertebral artery on movement of the head or neck. This is much less commonly diagnosed than previously and a regular relationship to head or neck movement must be confirmed before the diagnosis is acceptable. Where none of these causes can be established, the possibility of neck artery stenosis (almost always internal carotid) exists. This will be more likely if a carotid bruit can be detected on the affected side. Stenosis can be confirmed by angiography which may also show atheromatous plaque formation. This examination carries a significant risk of stroke and is only justifiable if there is prior agreement to do endarterectomy if the findings are of stenosis and/or plaque formation.

Clinical Features

These depend upon the territory involved. TIAs in the carotid system result in hemiparesis or monoparesis, dysphasia, unilateral sensory loss or paraesthesiae. Amaurosis fugax is a transient, unilateral, total or partial loss of vision lasting a few minutes. Fundoscopy may show an embolus (small pale body) traversing the retinal artery or one of its branches.

Vertebrobasilar TIAs are more varied. Common features are diplopia, facial numbness or paraesthesiae (especially in the circumoral area), vertigo, dysarthria and ataxia. Drop attacks may occur (*see* Chapter 3) but, without other focal neurological signs, it is probably unwise to attribute these to vertebrobasilar TIAs.

Likelihood of Stroke after TIA

Since a TIA indicates the existence of an abnormality in the cerebral circulation, there is an enhanced chance of stroke in TIA sufferers and if this occurs it is likely to be in the territory affected during the TIA. There is a clear time relationship between TIA and stroke, the latter being most likely in the 2 months after the TIA. Thereafter the risk decreases until by 6 months it is much the same as in the rest of the population of a similar age.

Carotid TIAs are much more likely to be followed by strokes, while vertebrobasilar TIAs are much more likely to recur yet less liable to lead to stroke.

Treatment of TIAs

In view of the likelihood of stroke after TIA (especially in the carotid territory), prophylaxis is advised. There is no conclusive evidence that warfarin should be given, but aspirin may have some beneficial effect. Its optimum dose is debatable, varying from 75 mg to 1200 mg daily. Because of the risk from intestinal bleeding, we advocate the lowest daily dose.

Where the vertebrobasilar TIAs are clearly associated with movements of the head and neck, a soft cervical collar should be supplied. Its main function is to remind patients to avoid unnecessary movement.

As indicated above, angiography may demonstrate carotid stenosis with or without atheromatous plaque formation. In these circumstances endarterectomy may be performed but this would rarely be considered in the UK in patients over 75 years.

SUMMARY AND CONCLUSION

Strokes are a common cause of death and severe prolonged disability bringing great misery to sufferers and their families.

Prevention is at present mainly a matter of detecting hypertension and effectively controlling it in younger age groups.

The assessment of the nature of disability in stroke is a complex matter involving the skills of doctor, nurse and therapists. A rational programme of rehabilitation can only be formulated after such full assessment.

The general practitioner and community nurses have a vital (and frequently incompletely exploited) role in helping to assess patients, in helping them to come to terms with permanent disability and in withstanding the rigours of an exhausting rehabilitation programme. Equally important is the general practitioner's role in supporting the families of stroke patients who frequently experience great stress and readily may feel extremely isolated and unsupported.

We have not discussed the question of when and whether stroke patients should be in hospital because this is so greatly affected by local circumstances, availability of geriatric beds, beds in stroke units and the degree of interest of local physicians and neurologists.

For the aged patient who is reasonably well supported at home and who sustains a severe stroke we would generally advocate retaining the patient at home on a 'wait and see' basis. It will usually be apparent within a few days whether the patient is going to succumb, stabilize or start to improve. At this stage (or earlier) the geriatrician should be asked for an opinion and he, together with the primary care team and family members, can decide what is best for the patient. For those who are likely to die quite soon it must surely be comforting in their more lucid moments to realize that they are in familiar surroundings and that the voices and faces around them are those of their own relations.

REFERENCES

Allison R. S. (1966) Perseveration as a sign of diffuse and focal brain damage. *Br. Med. J.* **2**, 1027, 1059.

Eaton-Griffith V. and Miller C. L. (1980) Volunteer stroke scheme for dysphasic patients with stroke. *Br. Med. J.* **281**, 1605.

Garraway W. M. (1976) In: *Stroke* (Gillingham F. J., Mawdsley C. and Williams A. E. eds). Edinburgh: Churchill Livingstone.

Kannel W. B., Wolf P. and Dawber T. R. (1978) Hypertension and cardiac impairments increase stroke risk. *Geriatrics* **33**, 71.

Marshall J. (1979) Differential diagnosis of stroke. *Adv. Neurol.* **25**, 177.

Oxbury J. M., Greenhall R. C. D. and Granger K. M. R. (1975) Predicting the outcome of stroke after cerebral infarction. *Br. Med. J.* **3**, 125.

7 DRUGS AND SAFER PRESCRIBING

INTRODUCTION

The elderly are by far the largest consumers of prescribed drugs, taking more than half of all drugs supplied within the National Health Service. About three-quarters of the over 75s receive prescribed medication with two-thirds of the recipients taking one to three drugs and the rest taking four or more. This age group is still increasing rapidly so the absolute numbers of persons having prescribed drugs is also increasing.

We wish to outline some known facts about drug use and the pharmacology of old age and try to offer some practical advice on good prescribing.

It has already been emphasized that many old people have multiple illnesses and complaints, many are the victims of social and financial stress which may give rise to somatic symptoms and frequently they have anxious and somewhat guilty relatives who insist that 'something must be done'. Faced with this scenario, it is understandably tempting for the doctor to reach for his prescription pad—an action which may be encouraged by subtle and occasionally unscrupulous promotional activities by pharmaceutical firms. This can readily lead to undesirable polypharmacy with risks of adverse effects, drug interactions and poor compliance.

It seems that many doctors believe that patients expect a prescription for every symptom. One study contradicts this notion since only 30–50 per cent of patients had this expectation, while 80–90 per cent of their doctors believed that a drug was being sought (Stimson, 1976).

Several studies have been made of prescribing patterns for older patients and it is known that about 85 per cent of the over 65s receive at least one drug regularly which is twice the proportion for the whole population. In one general practice study, half the 70+ group was receiving long-term therapy, mostly for heart disease, depression or anxiety. In 14 per cent of those on long-term therapy, there was no recorded contact with the general practitioner for 6 months or longer.

Diuretics and other 'heart drugs' were most commonly prescribed with analgesics (including non-steroidal anti-inflammatory drugs) and psychotropics close behind. Benzodiazepines were often prescribed for reasons which were not at all clear.

Another study of medication after discharge from hospital showed that one-fifth of patients had not been in touch with their general practitioner within a month of discharge and most seemed to have reverted, for better or for worse, to their preadmission drug regimes.

SOME PHARMACOLOGICAL CONSIDERATIONS

It is customary to consider these under the headings of pharmaco-kinetics and pharmacodynamics. 'Pharmacokinetics' is the term used to describe the way in which a drug is handled by the body, while 'pharmacodynamics' refers to the effect of a drug on physiological or pathological processes, i.e. the response to the drug. Both these aspects of drug action are significantly affected by ageing.

PHARMACOKINETICS OF AGEING

At any age drug handling is affected by:
1. Absorption
2. Distribution
3. Metabolism
4. Excretion

Absorption

Drugs are usually absorbed from stomach and small intestine and many factors are involved, some being affected by ageing. There may be a reduction in blood supply to the absorptive areas. There is a reduction in numbers of epithelial cells which have slower turnover and a reduction in absorptive area associated with decreased height of intestinal villi. Both basal and maximal secretion of gastric hydro-chloric acid are reduced which results in raised pH and an alteration in ionization and solubility of some drugs. The occurrence of duo-denal diverticula with bacterial colonization may predispose to malabsorption.

Despite the fact that some of these changes are common in old age, it seems that drug absorption is rarely significantly altered.

One important danger is from drug interaction which is more likely to occur in old age because of the frequency of multiple drug con-sumption. Tetracyclines will be converted to insoluble compounds if given along with salts of heavy metals such as iron, aluminium, calcium or magnesium. Drugs such as metoclopramide which speed up stomach emptying and hence speed the transit of drugs across the absorptive area may lead to reduced absorption, while drugs which delay stomach emptying will increase absorption (propantheline and many antidepressants with powerful anticholinergic effects). Thus a patient on digoxin for control of atrial fibrillation and who has been stabilized on a daily dose of 0·125 mg may escape from control if subsequently given metoclopramide and go back into cardiac failure.

Distribution

As shown in *Fig.* 7.1, body composition changes considerably with age.

This figure shows that specific gravity declines, the proportion of fat is increased and water decreases. Lean body mass is reduced from 25 per cent to 17 per cent. All these changes may significantly alter drug distribution. The reduction in body water causes reduction of volume of distribution of water-soluble drugs such as antipyrine, ethanol and paracetamol. On the other hand, the increase in body fat may result in increased volume of distribution of such lipid-soluble substances as diazepam and lignocaine. Some anaesthetic gases and short-acting barbiturates used in anaesthesia are highly fat soluble

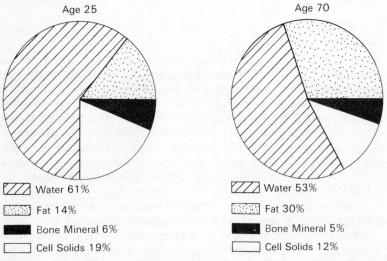

Fig. 7.1. Body composition in relation to age.

and this results in a prolonged postoperative recovery period as the drug is progressively released from solution.

It is difficult to quantify the precise effects of these age-related changes but, in general, they tend to produce higher plasma levels and longer plasma half-lives for many commonly used drugs. The consequences of changes in distribution may, however, often be compensated for by increased speed of metabolism and excretion.

Protein Binding of Drugs

In healthy old age there is no significant decrease in plasma proteins but in many old patients with multiple illnesses and poor nutritional status, proteins may be considerably lowered. This is especially so where liver function is affected as in congestive cardiac failure or primary liver disease.

Many commonly used drugs are highly bound to plasma protein and so changes in protein levels may alter their pharmacokinetics since only the unbound fraction is pharmacologically active. Where protein levels are low (especially the albumin fraction), fewer binding sites are available and the effect of a drug may thus be significantly increased.

Drugs vary greatly in their binding power and when a patient has been stabilized on a lightly binding drug such as tolbutamide, the addition of a powerful binder, such as a salicylate or phenothiazine, may displace the tolbutamide and thus predispose to dangerous hypoglycaemia. Likewise a patient on warfarin who later receives indomethacin or chloral may be in danger of excess anticoagulant effect from the rapid increase in bioavailable warfarin.

While the effects of competition for binding sites may be important for patients of all ages, they are particularly so in older patients, first because they are more likely to receive more than one drug and secondly because they are liable to have lowered protein levels and hence the competition becomes fiercer.

Metabolism

The liver is the organ most concerned with drug metabolism. Many drugs undergo a two-stage process. Stage I is reduction, oxidation or hydrolysis and is achieved by the activity of microsomal enzymes. Stage II is conjugation of the stage I metabolite usually with sulphuric or glucuronic acid to yield a soluble substance readily excreted by the kidneys. The enzymes involved in stage I are of low specificity and an enzyme induced in response to one drug will often be active in the metabolism of another drug. Some drugs have a much greater enzyme-inducing effect than others. Hence if two drugs are given together, one a powerful inducer and the other not, then there exists a danger that if the powerful inducer is withdrawn, the speed of metabolism of the other may be greatly reduced, leading to higher plasma levels and half-life. Thus where a patient who has been stabilized on a dose of a tricyclic antidepressant (lower inducing power) is then given a phenothiazine (higher inducing power), the tricyclic may be more rapidly metabolized and its therapeutic effect reduced or lost. Conversely a patient stabilized on a combination of a tricyclic plus phenothiazine may be in danger of tricyclic toxicity should the second drug be withdrawn. We have seen a similar danger where a patient on warfarin is admitted to hospital and a few days later manifests haemorrhagic tendencies because the previous regular and unsuspected alcohol consumption has been stopped.

To make things even more complex, some drugs are enzyme inhibitors, e.g. the H_2 antagonist cimetidine. Its use with other drugs may lead to increased enzyme levels. Thus the patient on a stable tolbutamide regime may be in danger of hypoglycaemia should cimetidine be added. Aspirin may also inhibit tolbutamide metabolism and steroids have the same effect on nortriptyline.

The liver is affected by age changes, decreasing in weight by more than a quarter between the third decade and 70 years. This results in significant reduction in hepatocytes, blood flow and enzyme activity. These changes may lead to reduced metabolism of such drugs as chlordiazepoxide, theophylline and nortriptyline.

Drugs with a high first-pass extraction (i.e. those which are so quickly extracted by the liver that significant proportions of an oral dose will be removed during the drug's first passage through the liver in the portal venous system) may show marked reductions in this extraction with age. Such drugs are chlormethiazole, labetalol, lignocaine and possibly other beta-adrenergic blocking substances. The bioavailability of these drugs may therefore be considerably increased in old age.

Excretion

Some drugs such as digitoxin are mainly excreted via the biliary tract, but the large majority are excreted via the kidneys by either glomerular filtration (digoxin, aminoglycoside antibiotics) or tubular secretion (penicillin and procainamide).

Kidney function was one of the first functions to be studied in relation to age and a linear decrease commences in the fourth or fifth decade and continues throughout life. Thus glomerular filtration falls by about 50 per cent between 20 and 90 years and renal blood flow falls by about the same amount. Tubular secretion declines by about 1 per cent per year from age 40 onwards so that this function will be reduced to 60 per cent of its former level at age 80 due to age changes alone. It is believed that these decrements are due to an age-related loss of nephrons; those which remain continue to function normally. In many old people, of course, these reductions will be aggravated by disease such as prostatism in males and infections or nephrosclerosis in both sexes. Hence many patients in their 80s may have lost 60 per cent to 80 per cent of their maximal renal function and while they may cope reasonably well normally, any stress such as a febrile illness with dehydration or a nephrotoxic drug will rapidly lead to uraemia and further renal damage. These patients have a marked reduction in capacity to excrete drugs.

Several studies have been made of digoxin excretion in relation to creatinine clearance and it is established that where clearance is less than 30 ml/min a dose of 0·25 mg will prove toxic. Hence 0·125 mg should generally be regarded as the safe maintenance dose for many very old patients (80+) or even in younger ones in poor general health and with multiple diseases. Very rarely where clearance is less than 10 ml/min, 0·0625 mg may be the appropriate maintenance dose. Most clinical laboratories can now perform plasma digoxin assays and once it is thought that a steady state has been achieved, any doubts about dosage may be dispelled by finding this level. Plasma half-life of digoxin is increased by about 40 per cent between young adulthood and the eighth decade.

While renal function can most accurately be measured by creatinine clearance, this is very difficult to perform in general practice (and may be difficult even in elderly patients in a hospital setting). Urea levels may be misleading since normal or slightly raised readings may occur in patients with considerable renal impairment. Serum creatinine levels provide a more sensitive guide.

Penicillin and its analogues are excreted almost entirely via the renal tubules, their plasma half-lives being almost doubled in old age. Thus higher concentrations of the drug are maintained for longer periods on similar doses to each other which may be advantageous to patients from their enhanced bactericidal effects. This, however, is far from being the case with aminoglycosides such as streptomycin and gentamicin, where the reduced glomerular excretion may readily lead to dangerously high plasma levels and serious 8th nerve damage with deafness or ataxia.

Some drugs share a common transport route within the tubules and if given simultaneously they may compete for available channels leading to plasma build-up. Examples are thiazide diuretics, sulphonylureas and the penicillins, two or more of which may quite commonly be prescribed at the same time.

Although some researchers have advocated the use of nomograms to assess renal function for younger patients, these may be misleading in sick aged patients with changes due to age plus past (and present) disease.

It should also be remembered that acute illness may result in sudden dramatic decrease in renal clearance, e.g. in acute myocardial infarction, respiratory tract infection or diarrhoea and vomiting or as a result of the nephrotoxic effects of a drug. In these circumstances a previously well-tolerated dose of a drug such as digoxin may rapidly become toxic.

These considerations lead us to suggest the following prescribing options:

1. The dose should be scaled down in line with renal function as assessed by age and clinical status. A serum creatinine level may be helpful. The dose decided upon should be given at usual intervals.
2. Another option is to use a 'normal' dose but extend the interval between doses.
3. Where renal function is very much reduced, the dose may have to be reduced and the intervals lengthened.

A useful guide to renal function may be obtained by noting the speed with which a patient corrects a raised plasma urea after a bout of dehydration. If, for example, an old lady is found to have a urea of 25–30 mmol/l when dehydrated during an acute illness but, on rehydration, reduces it to near normal in the space of a few days, this suggests that her renal reserves are not too reduced. This, of course, does not help with the current illness, but it is worth noting in her records for future reference.

PHARMACODYNAMICS

This has already been defined as the measurement of response of the body, or a pathological process to drug action.

Many studies have shown pharmacodynamic changes associated with ageing and related to altered receptor or tissue sensitivity. Thus the ageing central nervous system is considerably more sensitive to the effects of barbiturates and opiates, as shown by studies in which plasma levels are kept constant. This could be due to (or contributed to) by increase in permeability of the blood–brain barrier. One study (Castleden *et al.* 1977) showed that old people receiving 10 mg of nitrazepam at night showed significantly more psychomotor disturbance than did younger subjects with similar plasma levels. This impairment was also found to persist for 36 hours. Other changes in

drug response which appear not to be dependent upon pharmacokinetic effects are the greater effects of coumarin anticoagulants on
clotting factor synthesis in old age and the increased body sway and
reaction time with temazepam and chlormethiazole as well as the
increased nervous system depression with diazepam.

Another age-related pharmacodynamic alteration is the increased
drug effect on several homeostatic mechanisms, including baro-
receptor function in the maintenance of blood pressure. The efficiency
of thermoregulation may be reduced in old age and the addition of a
tranquillizer (major or minor) or the consumption of alcohol may
result in a real danger from hypothermia. Likewise the homeostatic
and autonomic mechanisms involved in blood sugar control and
bladder function may become precarious in old age and be associated
with greater sensitivity to drug effects.

From the foregoing sections on pharmacokinetics and pharmacodynamics it will be apparent that these are extremely complex issues
and the practical significance of some of them is debatable. What is
not in doubt, however, are the importance of reduced renal clearance
and the decrease in first-pass removal which may lead to marked
increase in bioavailability of some commonly used drugs.

ADVERSE DRUG REACTIONS

Advancing years carry an increased risk of unwanted and potentially
dangerous reactions to drugs. Many studies have shown that about
one in six elderly patients admitted to hospital are suffering from
adverse reactions at that time. One study involved 1998 patients aged
65 or more who were investigated at the time of admission to a British
department of geriatric medicine. There were 248 patients with
adverse reactions and 312 drugs were implicated. In the great majority
only one drug was involved, but in 59 two drugs were responsible and
in 5 cases, three drugs (Williamson and Chopin, 1980).

Figure 7.2 shows the numbers of reactions associated with the most
commonly used drugs.

Diuretics were the commonest cause of adverse reactions (60) with
psychotropics a close second.

Figure 7.3, however, gives a quite different picture since it shows
the proportion of adverse reactions among patients taking each drug
group.

Diuretics are relatively 'safe', while psychotropics, tremor and
rigidity controllers (anti-parkinsonian drugs) and hypotensives carry
the highest risk.

Adverse reactions increased significantly with increasing numbers
of drugs being taken; in patients receiving only one drug the rate was

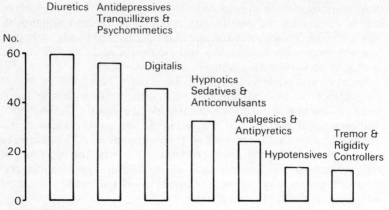

Fig. 7.2. Number of adverse reactions to commonly prescribed drugs.

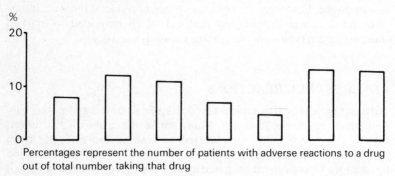

Percentages represent the number of patients with adverse reactions to a drug out of total number taking that drug

Fig. 7.3. Relative risk of adverse reactions with different drug groups.

10·8 per cent, while in those receiving six drugs the prevalence was 27·0 per cent, a highly significant difference.

An indication of the cost of adverse reactions to the Health Service is offered by the fact that in 209 patients the reaction was considered to have contributed to the need for hospital admission; in 55 it was the sole cause and in 154 contributory. Extrapolation of these figures to UK admissions rates to geriatric wards would suggest that, at the time of the survey (1976), adverse reactions may have been the sole cause for admission in 4000 cases and a contributory cause in about another 11 000.

Another alarming finding was that many patients never made a full recovery after adverse reactions. This does not necessarily mean that the adverse reaction *per se* was irreversible, but rather that the patient never regained his/her previous levels of function and independence. Overall, full recovery took place in 69 per cent of patients with reactions but for anti-parkinsonian drugs this proportion was only 46 per cent. Digitalis preparations, while quite likely to cause reactions, were relatively 'clean', having an 80 per cent chance of full patient recovery to previous levels.

Our readers will surely agree that these figures make sombre reading and emphasize the need for extreme caution in the use of drugs for old patients.

Illustrative Case

Mrs H. McD. had suffered from osteoarthritis of the right hip for many years. She also had sustained a minor left hemiparesis and suffered from mild dementia. At the age of 84, she was referred to the geriatric service for rehabilitation and was admitted to the assessment unit.

She complained bitterly of hip pain, and was given a non-steroidal anti-inflammatory drug in addition to the paracetamol which had been prescribed for many years.

Mrs H. McD. disliked being in hospital, saying that it was an erosion of her freedom, and refused to attend for physiotherapy. She also refused food, which the ward staff considered to be part of her 'protest'.

Ten days after admission, she vomited a large quantity of fresh blood and passed copious melaena stool. In spite of resuscitative measures, she developed renal failure and died. Post-mortem revealed a large, acute duodenal ulcer.

Although this lady had never presented dyspeptic symptoms, she had been difficult to assess, and upper gastrointestinal symptoms which she may have developed after administration of the non-steroidal anti-inflammatory drugs were misunderstood by the hospital staff.

Great care must be taken in prescribing this group of drugs to elderly people, who are particularly vulnerable to their adverse reactions, and who may not suffer the typical symptoms of peptic ulceration.

COMPLIANCE WITH PRESCRIBER'S INSTRUCTIONS

It has been pointed out that when one acquires a new car or camera, one is supplied with elaborate and carefully composed booklets of instructions containing photographs and diagrams to ensure proper understanding and usage. Drugs are now most carefully researched, elaborately tested in animals and thereafter in extensive clinical trials. In short, every step is taken to ensure the greatest possible safety. Yet patients may thereafter be given prescriptions for these drugs and obtain them from the pharmacist with little or no notion of what they are for and usually no idea of possible ill effects. Recognition of this weak link in the chain of events from manufacture to consumption is now widespread and many doctors (including general practitioners) have been trying to achieve improvements.

Most old people in the community are responsible for their own medication. Various studies have shown that about three-quarters make errors, some potentially very serious. Patients most likely to have compliance problems are the very old (85+), those living alone and those who are confused. There is a high correlation between poor compliance and cognitive impairment. The more drugs being taken and the more complex the regime, the greater is the chance of poor compliance. Inadequate efforts at explanation may be compounded by hearing difficulties and poor vision will reduce the value of written instructions—especially if the writing is small or indistinct. There is no justification for the use of such largely meaningless rubrics as 'as before' or 'as directed'.

Illustrative Case

Mrs M. D., aged 76, had been admitted to the geriatric unit suffering from acute confusion and immobility. She had sustained a myocardial infarct, with rapid atrial fibrillation and congestive cardiac failure. She was a non-insulin-dependent diabetic.

On recovery, she demonstrated very mild mental impairment and coped reasonably well on a home visit with the occupational therapist. The team were anxious, however, about her ability to cope with her drugs: digoxin, a diuretic and two oral hypoglycaemic agents. She was given a Dosett, which is a plastic box divided up into 28 compartments—4 per day for a week, which may act as an aid to drug compliance. The district nurse was recruited to fill this each week.

Four days after discharge home, a call came in to the geriatric service from the general practitioner, saying that Mrs M. D. had become acutely confused during the previous night. By the time the geriatrician visited, she was alert, but described symptoms compatible with hypoglycaemia during the early hours of the morning. On close inspection of her drugs, it emerged that not only was she taking the pills from the Dosett, she was also taking them from the traditional containers, which had been left alongside! Once this error had been explained to her and the bottles removed to a cupboard, she coped well with no further confusional episodes. She liked her 'gadget', but, in retrospect, she would have been managed better with a conventional approach and clear instructions.

Errors in compliance which have been identified include:

1. Failure to take the drug due to either misunderstanding of

instructions or inability to obtain the drug, e.g. patient house-bound and no one to take prescription to chemist.

2. Self-medication with 'across the counter' drugs, or drugs left over from a previous illness. The former occurrence is maybe more likely to happen now that there is a limited list of drugs prescribable under NHS regulations. Sometimes a patient may be taking drugs prescribed for another person such as a spouse or a 'helpful' neighbour.

3. Inaccurate timing and spacing of doses.

4. Mistaking one drug for another, e.g. taking digoxin thrice daily and potassium supplements only once.

Factors which may Impair Compliance

The following factors may contribute to impairing compliance:

Failing vision; poor hearing
Poor memory; dementia
Unfamiliarity with modern medications
Failure to understand instructions
Unsuitable packaging (blister packs, child proofing, etc.)

For the patient with poor vision or deafness it is necessary to take extra care to ensure comprehension—large, printed instructions on a separate card, or the involvement of a third party as supervisor (in which case it is essential to ensure that this person receives full and accurate appraisal).

Where memory is failing, and particularly where the patient is dementing, the first requirement is to be aware of this failure and methods of detecting these conditions are outlined in Chapter 2. Where significant dementia is established, the only foolproof way of ensuring compliance is to enlist the help of a reliable third person.

Problems can easily arise over the use of generic and proprietary names. Thus a patient who has become accustomed to receive medication labelled 'propranolol' is entitled to feel unsure when the next supply is called 'Inderal'. Manufacturers ought to be careful to avoid similar sounding names for products. We have seen a near disaster when a patient who was supposed to receive 'tryptophan' received instead 'Triptafen'. It will be very surprising if this particular error does not recur.

A study of elderly patients after discharge from hospital showed that nearly half had not conformed with hospital instructions on medication and had not seen their general practitioner. Many, indeed, had reverted to the medication they had been taking prior to admission.

Improving Compliance

The simpler the regime, the better the compliance will be. Therefore, make it as simple as possible; this may mean transgressing the golden rule of therapeutic purists that combined preparations should not be used. Wherever possible, no more than three drugs should be prescribed. The minimum number of daily doses should be sought, using whatever preparation allows this (despite the fact that slow release formulations may be more expensive). Relating dosage to mealtimes, bedtime and rising time often may help.

Instructions should be clearly printed on a card and in some instances, sample tablets or capsules should be stuck on the card with Sellotape or a similar device. Clear glass containers should be used (except, of course, where light has to be excluded) with ordinary or winged-screw tops. Where the patient is attending hospital (as day patient or outpatient), he/she should be given a medication card on which the general practitioner or hospital doctor can note any changes of medication. We try to ensure that day patients bring all their current medication with them at each attendance. This enables the day-hospital staff to check what they are receiving and, where indicated, tablet counts can be done to ascertain how many have been consumed since the last attendance.

The use of various dispensing devices such as Dosett boxes with several separate compartments for each day of the week has achieved only limited acceptance. Family members sometimes display notable ingenuity and resourcefulness as in the case of the dementing old lady with parkinsonism on a rather complex régime of Madopar and bromocriptine. Her family undertook to visit her several times each day and to lay out her medication in egg cups. Each egg cup had a clockface alongside with an indication of when it should be used. The first visitor in the morning was her son-in-law on his way to work and a potential gap in supervision in the afternoon was overcome by a phone call from her daughter to remind her of her mid-afternoon medication.

Small tablets go down more easily than large because some old people have poor salivary flow and difficulty in swallowing larger tablets. Adequate amounts of water or other beverage should be ordered with medication, e.g. a whole cupful of water will increase the chance of rapid transit to the stomach and diminish the risk of prolonged contact with the buccal or oesophageal mucosa and serious ulceration as may occur with emepronium bromide or Slow K. Old people often prefer liquid or dispersible preparations, especially when acutely ill, dehydrated or drowsy from any cause. Measuring vessels for liquid preparations are much superior to spoons especially where there is arthritis, tremor or poor vision. It should be remembered that suppositories are useful, especially for such drugs as aminophylline, chlorpromazine, some non-steroidal anti-inflammatory drugs and morphine. Inhalation therapy generally requires good mental function and the ability to coordinate inspiration with the manually operated trigger release. A nebulizer may be very helpful in some patients but may be poorly tolerated by confused and restless patients.

Many old people have difficulty in making their way to the doctor's premises especially in inclement weather and primary teams should make efforts to identify these patients and make special provision for them. This group includes the most aged, those with locomotor or stroke disabilities and those with dementia. Wherever possible, family members of such patients should receive advice and instruction on medication for their elders including details of each drug, dosage and possible side-effects. Where no such family support is available, someone from primary care should be entrusted with regular visiting and checking.

REPEAT PRESCRIPTIONS

Between half and three-quarters of all prescriptions issued for old patients are on a 'repeat prescription' basis. Surveys have revealed widely differing policies with regard to this practice; some elderly patients on quite complex drug regimes may see no one from primary care for months on end, while other general practitioners will not countenance repeat prescriptions at all and will instead give a 3 months' supply of drugs after which each patient is seen and his/her medication reviewed. It would seem that the latter arrangement is the one to be aimed at for all patients (and not just the old).

The proportion of drugs supplied on repeat prescriptions rises with the age of the patient. Some 5 per cent of these prescriptions have been shown to contain errors and estimates have been made which suggest that 10 per cent are, in any case, unnecessary.

The conditions for which repeat prescriptions are most frequently issued are cardiovascular (diuretics, digoxin and hypotensives), musculoskeletal conditions (analgesics and non-steroidal anti-inflammatory drugs), insomnia and anxiety/depression (psychotropics and antidepressants).

SOME SPECIAL PROBLEMS IN PRESCRIBING FOR ELDERLY PATIENTS

We wish now to deal with common problems encountered with different drug groups which we have found to be frequently associated with misunderstandings.

Digoxin

This is a commonly prescribed drug in old age and it can readily cause adverse reactions which may be unrecognized or misdiagnosed as some other condition. Digoxin toxicity in old patients commonly presents as confusion and general loss of well-being without the characteristic nausea and vomiting. Any old person receiving a digitalis preparation who becomes vaguely unwell should be strongly suspected of having intoxication and, where possible, a plasma assay performed. This is now available in most clinical laboratories. It should be remembered that the blood sample should not be with-drawn until at least 6 hours after the last oral dose.

It is certain that until quite recently many old patients received digoxin unnecessarily and studies have shown that about 4 out of 5 patients on digoxin therapy came to no harm when the drug was stopped. It seems therefore that in the absence of uncontrolled atrial fibrillation or firm evidence of paroxysmal supraventricular tachy-cardia, there is little or no indication for digoxin therapy. It is true that its inotropic effect upon heart muscle will benefit a few patients in sinus rhythm, but it is not possible to identify them in advance and since the large majority will not be benefited, we make it our policy to restrict digoxin use to the above two categories. Digoxin dosage has already been discussed in relation to excretion.

Initiation of digoxin therapy usually requires a loading dose of 0·50 mg to 0·75 mg which we prefer to give as 0·25 mg twice on day 1 and 0·25 mg on day 2, response being assessed by changes in pulse and apex rates. It is probably wise not to give larger single doses than 0·25 mg in case the patient has unusual sensitivity to the drug in which case very unpleasant gastric irritation may occur.

In recent years we have witnessed an encouraging reduction in cases of digoxin intoxication. This has happened quite suddenly and is in marked contrast to 1977 when one of us encountered 4 cases in 1 week. We feel that the pendulum may have swung rather too far and we are now encountering patients who require digoxin but who have never received sufficient to produce therapeutic levels.

There is no place for the old practice of giving digoxin 0·25 mg daily for 5 days with a 'holiday' at weekends. This is illogical and likely to result in poorer compliance. The proper daily dose should be determined and taken regularly.

Diuretics

Diuretics are among the most commonly prescribed drugs for old people in the UK. These are extremely valuable and powerful weapons in the fight against illness and have certainly been responsible for a great improvement in the comfort and ease of many who would otherwise have died slowly and in distress. One of us is old enough to remember the era preceding powerful oral diuretics when we had to rely upon injections of organic mercurials of meagre diuretic potency and associated with serious risks of renal damage and exfoliative dermatitis.

It may be that the ease of ridding a patient of excess tissue fluid with modern diuretics has made us less aware of just how powerful these drugs really are. It is an easy step from this *blasé* attitude to their overuse.

Many old people have diminished mobility due to arthritis, obesity, dyspnoea or sometimes just laziness! Some will respond by sitting all day in their chairs. Some old women may even sit up all night as well. The result is often oedema of the lower extremities which will be aggravated by chronic venous insufficiency due to previous venous thrombosis or varicose veins.

Gravitational oedema of this type is by far the commonest cause of lower limb oedema in old age and by itself it is not an indication for long-term diuretic use. In mild cases, all that is necessary is firm advice to move about more and to use a footstool. If the patient habitually has an afternoon nap, then she should be encouraged to lie down on her bed or sofa for this purpose. Raising the foot of the bed may help, as will the use of a rocking chair which encourages the pumping action of calf muscles without any conscious extra effort by the patient. Perhaps families should be encouraged to view a rocking chair as a suitable eightieth birthday present? Where the oedema is more marked, a diuretic may be prescribed for a few days till the excess fluid has disappeared after which the simple measures outlined above may prevent its recurrence. Where a diuretic is thought to be necessary on a continuing basis, it will rarely be needed 7 days per week. Support stockings are prescribable under the NHS and often provide excellent control of gravitational oedema.

The commonest adverse reactions associated with diuretics are hypokalaemia and postural hypotension. Less often hyponatraemia may occur and sometimes serious depletion of extracellular fluid may result with a potentially fatal outcome. Recently attention has been drawn to the occurrence of hypomagnesaemia which, if unrecognized and uncorrected, may lead to great difficulty in correcting simultaneous hypokalaemia.

There is argument in relation to younger age groups as to whether routine potassium supplements are necessary in patients receiving potassium-losing diuretics. In old age there is already a tendency towards low potassium status both because of relatively low intake and possible impairment of renal potassium conservation. We therefore advise that all elderly patients on potassium-wasting diuretics should receive supplementation. While there is a place for potassium-sparing diuretics, we have been impressed by the frequency with which we have seen dangerous hyperkalaemia in patients on these drugs (and also occasionally a paradoxical hypokalaemic patient). We are aware, of course, that we tend to see only the 'bad cases' and there must be many old people who are safely treated with these drugs.

Speed of action of diuretics should always be considered. Loop diuretics such as frusemide and bumetanide act very rapidly and hence may cause problems such as retention of urine in males with prostatic hypertrophy. In both sexes, where there is detrusor instability the sudden rapid flow of urine may cause the patient to get 'caught short', especially where mobility is poor and the patient may not have time to get to the toilet. Even relatively fit old people with good mobility and agility may find that these drugs interfere with their daily routine. Old ladies may not care to venture out shopping till the first 4- or 5-hour brisk diuresis is over. Hence we recommend that the first choice should be a thiazide diuretic (which is also much cheaper). Where the patient is in severe congestive cardiac failure, a loop diuretic should be used initially but it should be explained to the patient that a very brisk diuresis is to be expected and there may be incontinence. The patient who has been warned of this and appreciates that a brisk diuresis is a good sign will be much less upset than the patient who, for the first time in her adult life, finds herself unable to control her bladder.

Hypotensive Agents

It has been emphasized above that hypotensive drugs were among those most likely to cause adverse reactions. Where blood pressure is high and there are clinical consequences such as angina or evidence of left ventricular strain, then it is necessary to bring down the pressure, but even in such clear-cut circumstances it should be done gradually and with caution since sudden reduction may be dangerous.

Patients on long-term thiazide therapy for hypertension should have regular tests for glycosuria and hyperglycaemia.

Beta-blocking drugs should be avoided where there is a history of cardiac failure or when the patient has chronic obstructive airways disease. These drugs may have other undesirable side-effects such as bradycardia, postural hypotension, cold extremities and marked lethargy and fatigue.

There is growing evidence that calcium antagonists such as nifedipine are effective in treating hypertension and appear to have fewer serious side-effects.

Angiotensin-converting enzyme inhibitors such as captopril are now widely used in the treatment of hypertension, especially in North America, but their benefits and dangers in the elderly are not yet clear. It is known, however, that they must be used very cautiously in older patients with low starting doses otherwise there is a risk of severe hypotension.

Psychotropic Drugs

This group of drugs is undoubtedly overprescribed for all adult ages and certainly so for older patients. It has already been shown that they carry a high risk of adverse reactions. We have the impression that where in earlier times a placebo would have been prescribed, the modern doctor may be more apt to prescribe a psychotropic drug.

Hypnotics

It is customary to blame general practitioners for careless over-prescribing of hypnotics especially for older patients. This is frequently unfair and several studies have shown that many old people are started on hypnotics while in hospital and led to expect this medication when they return home. It seems that the nightly 'sedative round' is not yet a thing of the past in hospital although it may be less formalized. Another relevant fact is that sleep problems in some old people are well nigh insoluble.

It is singularly unfortunate that nature tends to allocate less sleep as we grow older despite the fact that many old people find that time hangs heavily and, being understimulated and underoccupied, may seek solace and escape in 'natural' sleep. When denied this, they (or their relatives) may demand 'unnatural' sleep. The problem is often compounded by the fact that many tend to sleep during the day and this eats into their 'ration' of hours of sleep so that they are wakeful at night. In extreme cases, especially in dementia, patients turn night into day and are up and active all night with disastrous effects upon carers. Sanford (1975) showed that, of all the stresses which old people may inflict upon their families, the least supportable was disturbed nights. This is not surprising and common sense suggests that while ordinary people can cope with great demands if adequately rested, if denied this, they will rapidly collapse.

The quality of sleep is altered with age; old people have more difficulty and take longer to fall asleep. While a young adult may take only a few minutes to go to sleep, an old person may take a half-hour. The old also have many more wakeful intervals—up to seven per night by age 75 compared to two in young adults. The deep sleep associated with slow-wave activity on an electroencephalogram is markedly reduced in the elderly, while REM sleep (i.e. that associated with rapid eye movements) is either not affected or only slightly reduced. The sleep induced by hypnotics is not the same as natural sleep, for example the amount of REM sleep is much reduced. In consequence after 8 hours of sedative-induced sleep the patient may feel less refreshed than after 5 or 6 hours of natural slumber.

Thus nature and custom combine to make a problem of sleeplessness in old age, one which is commonly deposited in the lap of the general practitioner with demands for sleeping pills.

The first requirement is to find out if there is any associated cause for the insomnia, such as dyspnoea, pain from osteoarthritis (or other musculoskeletal condition), erythrocyanosis, severe constipation with impacted rectum, leg cramps, 'restless legs' and troublesome dysuria or urinary retention with overflow and nocturia. Simple inquiry will generally reveal the existence of such conditions. Patient and relatives should be asked if there is any source of anxiety such as unpaid bills or fear of vandals (in large housing estates especially). The possibility of depression must be borne in mind and inquiry along the lines suggested in the appendix to Chapter 8 should be made.

Where nocturia is a factor, a bedside commode for females and a urinal for males will ease the problem and offer partial relief by minimizing the degree of disturbance to the patient and supporters. Restriction of evening fluid intake may also be beneficial.

Where there are no associated conditions, time should be spent in explanation that older people often require less sleep. Reassurance that this is normal may help patient and relatives to accept the condition more readily.

Where the patient is physically capable, regular exercise and participation in mental activity such as family games and recreation should be prescribed. Efforts should be made to reduce the amount of daytime napping. A warm milk drink at bedtime may help, but the oft-recommended alcoholic 'night cap' is not indicated since it induces sleep which is often followed by wakefulness and a troublesome diuresis with nocturia. A cosy bed in a warm room will often help the patient to fall asleep.

Once it has been decided to prescribe a sedative, it is advisable to indicate to the patient and carers that this will be for a limited period only—just long enough to see the patient through an emotional crisis, time of anxiety or intercurrent illness. The choice of drug is often difficult, partly because of the wide range to choose from. In general the long-acting substances such as flurazepam are to be avoided since they lead to hangover effects and deterioration in psychomotor function. The very short-acting benzodiazepines such as triazolam, on the other hand, are often associated with 'rebound insomnia' when withdrawn, and some patients on long-term therapy with these drugs may experience withdrawal effects in the afternoon or evening as the tissue concentrations fall to zero. We have found that chlormethiazole in a dose of 192 mg is a suitable sedative with no serious side-effects. Many doctors use chloral hydrate in a dose of 500 mg at night time and this is certainly a drug which has stood the test of time. Its derivative dichloralphenazone is less likely to cause gastric irritation and has a mild analgesic effect, which may be useful where there is pain or discomfort as in arthritis or after injury. It is, however, rather a large tablet which could prove difficult for old people to swallow so the liquid preparation may be preferred. In general, we prefer to avoid benzodiazepines but of those available within the NHS, temazepam (10 mg) and lormetazepam (1 mg) appear to have the most appropriate half-lives—neither too long nor too short.

Tranquillizers

The benzodiazepines are by far the most commonly prescribed minor tranquillizers, diazepam, lorazepam and chlordiazepoxide being the most popular. While of value for short-term use in anxiety states, they are now regarded as being moderately addictive and their long-term use should be avoided. It is often very difficult to wean patients off these drugs because of unpleasant withdrawal effects. Their half-life is increased in older patients—a useful guide is the patient's age in years. Occasionally patients may respond in a paradoxical fashion to these drugs with restlessness or even aggressiveness. Where there is marked anxiety such as after a burglary, diazepam 2 mg thrice daily may be helpful but, once again, it should be offered as a 2- or 3-week course and not as a permanent prop to patient and carers. Larger doses may cause drowsiness, unsteady gait and slurred speech and readily lead to falls.

In severe states of anxiety or in dementing patients with restlessness and wandering, phenothiazines or butyrophenones may be necessary. Our first choice would be thioridazine starting with 10 mg t.d.s. with some patients requiring rather larger doses such as 25 mg t.d.s. Dementia sufferers sometimes have a marked tendency to restlessness (and sometimes aggression) in the evening and it is highly desirable to try to pre-empt this by giving an extra dose about 4 p.m. If the excited restless state is allowed to occur, much larger doses may be required; the patient may then end up by being very drowsy and sleepy all next day only to wake up in the evening with even greater behaviour disturbance. It should be borne in mind that it is rarely necessary to continue phenothiazine therapy for prolonged periods since the patient often settles down and ceases to be a disturbance. Hence, after 2 or 3 weeks the dose should be reduced and often only the late-afternoon dose is required on a long-term basis.

For paranoid states, thioridazine is usually effective and it seems that these patients are often much more tolerant to major tranquillizers and may require much larger doses for effective control of symptoms. Nevertheless, the same caution should be exercised and a start made with 10 mg t.d.s. increasing until the desired effect is achieved. The drug may slowly accumulate in the patient's tissues resulting in drowsiness, unsteadiness, postural hypotension and mental confusion. Another undesirable effect is constipation, a condition from which many old people suffer and which may culminate in faecal impaction when a phenothiazine is added.

Where the patient is very excited and perhaps delirious, it may be necessary to use the intramuscular route, the dose then being about half the oral requirement.

All these drugs have powerful extrapyramidal effects and can produce drug-induced parkinsonism which may lead to serious problems of immobility and falls. Even after the drug is stopped this condition may persist for months. It is then likely to be diagnosed as idiopathic parkinsonism and the patient may then be committed unnecessarily to lifetime anti-parkinsonian therapy with all the attendant dangers.

Illustrative Case

Mr A. C. was a 78-year-old widower living in residential care. He was noticed to have a tremor of both hands and on a visit by the general practitioner to the home, Mr A. C. was mentioned. As a result he was referred to hospital as an outpatient to exclude Parkinson's disease. He was duly seen and was started on L -dopa therapy—Sinemet-110 q.i.d.—with instructions to double the dose 7 days later. However before this increase could take place, the general practitioner was called in as Mr A. C. had become very confused, especially at night, disturbing the other residents. He was treated with thioridazine 25 mg t.i.d. and his behaviour settled. After several weeks, Mr A. C.'s mobility was noticed to have deteriorated—a slow, shuffling gait—and he required help with dressing as he was very slow and having difficulty with buttons. His general practitioner felt that Mr A. C.'s parkinsonian features were increasing and doubled his dose of Sinemet. Subsequently he became confused again and chlorpromazine 25 mg q.i.d. was added to his drug regime. His general condition deteriorated rapidly and he became bedfast and totally dependent. He was referred to the local geriatric service who arranged his admission to the assessment unit. Within a week of stopping all his drugs Mr A. C. was mentally clear, independent in self-care and was found to have a senile tremor. He was fortunate that his symptoms of drug-induced parkinsonism resolved so quickly.

A growing problem is tardive dyskinesia following prolonged anti-psychotic drug therapy and it seems probable that more older patients will suffer from this distressing condition as a result of treatment in earlier life. It can be very disabling and response to treatment is generally unsatisfactory.

Antidepressants

A study of a random sample of old people in Edinburgh showed that 3–4 per cent of the men and 6–7 per cent of the women were suffering from depression (as diagnosed by the psychiatrist member of the research team). It is therefore a common problem and as it is an extremely unpleasant condition, general practitioners should be alert to its probability in older patients. It may appear in its classic fashion in the elderly, in which case it is easily diagnosed. However, sometimes it presents in a rather unusual fashion, one most important being the apparent aggravation of a pre-existing condition such as stroke, arthropathy or parkinsonism. Its detection may then be difficult since the deterioration may readily be ascribed to progression or relapse of the disease. Patients with parkinsonism often look depressed, their speech is flat, their movements are slow and their whole demeanour resembles that of a depressed patient and it may be very difficult to decide if there is a significant mood disturbance.

All team members are encouraged to be on the lookout for anything which might suggest depression. The nursing staff and therapists are generally with the patients for much more prolonged periods than the doctors so their observations are very important. Does the patient appear withdrawn, does she make significant remarks such as being a nuisance, 'better dead', etc.? Our general rule is that if any team member seriously considers depression to be present then we review the case in detail and if any doubt persists we arrange a careful trial of antidepressant therapy. In general practice this approach would include the community nurses, home helps, wardens of sheltered housing and, of course, family and neighbours in regular contact with the patient.

Antidepressants when effective are a great boon to elderly depressed patients in whom a good therapeutic response is to be regularly expected. Unfortunately, they also may cause serious adverse effects which, in some cases, may preclude their use and this may necessitate electroconvulsive therapy.

The original tricyclics—imipramine and amitriptyline—are as powerful as any newer drugs and many psychiatrists use them as first-line therapy in all cases. Unfortunately they also have powerful anticholinergic effects and many old people are highly susceptible to these. Common problems are dry mouth, blurred vision, constipation, postural hypotension and micturition disturbances (amounting sometimes to urinary retention, especially in males). Patients with chronic glaucoma, however, may safely take antidepressants as long as they continue to use their meiotic eye drops.

More recently introduced antidepressants are claimed to be less toxic and we believe that drugs such as mianserin and trazodone do cause fewer anticholinergic side-effects. We have often used them in old patients especially where their general condition is poor and it is suspected that homeostasis is inefficient. In all cases careful watch must be kept for drowsiness, confusion and postural hypotension both during the introduction of therapy and thereafter.

As with most other drugs, general practitioners should familiarize themselves with one or two antidepressants and stick with them until convinced by good evidence that others have distinct advantages; such evidence should not be based solely upon promotional literature and sales talk.

Patients on identical doses show very large variations in plasma levels. Some claim that there may be a tenfold variability in tricyclic plasma levels so it is essential to start with low doses and increase cautiously in order to obtain the optimum maintenance dose.

We recommend a starting dose of 25 mg of imipramine (or the equivalent of a newer drug). This will be increased to 50 mg after 4 or 5 days and then to 75 mg after a similar interval if there are no significant side-effects. This is the commonest maintenance dose in our patients and more than this, although sometimes needed, will often be poorly tolerated.

Where the first choice of antidepressant is ineffective (after a 4–6-week trial), another should be tried, preferably one with a different chemical effect. If this also is ineffective, then the diagnosis should be reviewed and if depression is confirmed a psychiatrist's opinion is sought and electroconvulsive therapy considered. Perhaps in general practice it would be a good rule to seek the help of the geriatrician or psychiatrist after the first drug has been ineffective.

SUMMARY AND CONCLUSION

We shall offer some guidance towards safer prescribing:

1. The first question to be posed should be: 'Is treatment necessary?' Hence accurate diagnosis is essential, based upon history and examination with a careful check of current (and recent) drug consumption. This is time-consuming for a busy general practitioner, but time spent initially getting the facts right may mean more time saved later on trying to clear up the mess! Thus before starting treatment for parkinsonism, it is

essential to check that there has been no use of major tranquillizers in the last few weeks or months, e.g. prochlorperazine for postural instability. The tremor of parkinsonism is characteristic, but senile tremor or even anxiety tremor may be mistaken for it by the unwary. Never prescribe a drug for falls or 'dizziness', but always try to find the cause and rectify it.

2. Is drug treatment really indicated? As already outlined, simple explanation and reassurance may be all that are necessary for alleged insomnia in old age. Where it is decided to prescribe a placebo, the temptation to 'go one better' and use the latest benzodiazepine should be firmly resisted. Why not offer 50 mg of ascorbic acid? Some old people may actually benefit from this, especially in winter and early spring when the usual sources of vitamin C are scarce and expensive.

3. Give as few drugs as possible and stick to tried favourites. Despite the contrary advice of some clinical pharmacologists, it may sometimes be appropriate to prescribe long-acting or combined preparations if this simplifies dosage regimes and improves compliance. Dosage at mealtimes and bedtime also may improve compliance. When adding extra drugs to a patient's regime, the British National Formulary (or equivalent) should be consulted to see if interactions are likely. Remember to ask about 'across-the-counter' medication since patients and relatives may not regard these as drugs at all and hence not mention their consumption.

4. Review drug regimes regularly and always when another drug is being added or when intercurrent illness occurs. Renal excretion may be reduced during acute illness and distribution or metabolism affected by adding another drug.

   It is good practice to review patients who have been on hypotensive therapy when they reach old age. We have seen a number of patients in whom a careful withdrawal of hypotensive drugs has been followed by no increase in blood pressure in spite of incontrovertible evidence of hypertension in earlier life.

5. Give clear instructions. It is worth while spending some time in explanation and making sure that the patient understands what the drug is for, its dosage and what untoward effects may occur. Where vision is poor, extra large clear printing should be used and where there is dementia some other person should be enrolled as supervisor—a daughter or son, home help or friendly neighbour. In these circumstances the supervisor must be fully and accurately informed.

6. Start with low doses. For highly toxic drugs and those with variable pharmacokinetic and pharmacodynamic effects (e.g.

tricyclic antidepressants), the initial dose should probably not exceed a quarter of the ordinary adult dose.

We conclude by reiterating that modern drugs carefully administered and supervised offer great benefit to elderly patients, and the doctor who takes the trouble to understand their pharmacokinetics and pharmacodynamics will derive great satisfaction from seeing the improvements resulting from his or her prescription.

REFERENCES

Castleden C. M., George C. M., Marcer D. *et al.* (1977) Increased sensitivity to nitrazepam in old age. *Br. Med. J.* **1**, 10.
Sanford J. R. A. (1975) Tolerance of debility in elderly dependents by supporters at home: its significance for hospital practice. *Br. Med. J.* **3**, 471.
Stimson G. V. (1976) Doctor–patient interaction and some problems for prescribing. *J. R. Coll. Gen. Pract.* **26**, suppl. 1, 88.
Williamson J. and Chopin J. M. (1980) Adverse reactions to prescribed drugs in the elderly: a multicentre investigation. *Age Ageing* **9**, 73.

8 PREVENTION, SCREENING AND CASE FINDING IN PRIMARY CARE

Until recently the prevailing view of old age as a time of loss and irrecoverable dependency meant that preventive action was rarely considered.

The remarkable successes of modern geriatric services, however, have helped to change this negative stereotype. Successful rehabilitation of old people after stroke or acute illness and in apparently unpromising circumstances has shown that partial or total restoration of independence is often possible. This new-found optimism led some workers to entertain ideas of prevention in relation to old age and considerable success has been achieved.

It must be admitted, however, that primary prevention of disease in old age can only have limited scope, since many of the serious common diseases such as atherosclerosis and some forms of cancer have their origins much earlier in life through poor diet, tobacco abuse and other environmental or behavioural factors. Other serious conditions such as Alzheimer-type dementia and parkinsonism are common in old age, yet we have no idea of their cause and hence their prevention is at present impossible.

Despite this, even in old age, good diet, regular exercise and avoidance of cigarette and alcohol abuse will help to preserve good health as will social measures such as adequate pensions, suitable housing and recreational facilities. Counselling in preparation for retirement will help older persons to cross safely the Rubicon which separates the economically active and 'worth-while' from the retired and 'burdensome' state of old age.

There is no doubt that many people now enter retirement with much greater optimism and determination to enjoy their remaining years than was the case a few decades ago, and surveys have shown that many in the 65–74 age group retain remarkable health and vigour and continue to enjoy their new-found leisure in a wide variety of ways. This is most encouraging and confirms that there is considerable scope for health education aimed at the whole community, the elderly and their families. This educative process must also be directed specifically at the medical and nursing professions who frequently harbour the most negative of all views of old age, based as they have been almost exclusively upon their hospital training.

It is to be hoped, therefore, that with greater public and professional awareness of the importance of health rather than disease there will be a continuing improvement in fitness as people enter the senium.

The benefits of primary prevention are mostly long term; short-term gains are likely to be rather few and unspectacular. However, other preventive activities may offer a much quicker and dramatic effect with improvements in levels of independence and, it is to be hoped, a more rational use of scarce resources (both health and social service). This brings us to a consideration of the terms *screening* and *case finding*.

SCREENING

Various definitions exist of the screening process, each with slightly different emphases but all imply the planned detection and reversal of precursors of disease (risk factors). The Department of Health and Social Security offered the following definition: 'Screening differs from ordinary clinical practice in that it involves seeking out people with no overt symptoms of disease and asking them to undergo examination and tests to see whether the condition to be identified is present' (DHSS, 1976). Risk factors which are commonly sought are asymptomatic hypertension, hypercholesterolaemia, cervical metaplasia, raised intraocular tension, etc.

This type of medical activity became very popular in the years after the Second World War especially in North America, where centres were established to carry out multiple screening procedures on apparently healthy individuals. This became known as multiphasic screening and has become a profitable commercial enterprise. After the multiphasic screening is completed, the person's primary physician is sent a report with the results of all tests and assays with an indication of which fall outside 'normality'. This physician is then expected to take all necessary steps to safeguard the patient's health including, if necessary, the removal or mitigation of any identified risk factor.

This all appears so rational and sensible that even to question it seems to some of its protagonists to be totally churlish. However, scientific proof of benefit does not exist nor has it been shown to be cost-effective. A London study was conducted under the auspices of Professor Walter Holland to answer essential questions about multiphasic screening (South-east London Screening Study Group, 1977).

Large numbers of individuals aged 45–64 were screened by enthusiastic general practitioners and their progress was compared with that of a control population who were not screened. There were no significant differences between the groups in respect of morbidity, mortality or use of resources. It is not known why screening of this sort has not proved to be effective, but one argument is that the main deficiency was a failure by the general practitioners involved in the London study to take appropriate action with regard to identified risk factors. This excuse is a gross oversimplification and does not stand up to scrutiny. Thus, if a self-selected group of general practitioners who are enthusiastic enough to cooperate in such a research scheme could not make it successful, it is most unlikely that 'ordinary' general practitioners would be more effective.

The results of this study were taken seriously by health authorities and the outcome was that it was decided not to provide multiphasic population screening within the National Health Service, although some private and commercial organizations offer a service to individuals and to industrial concerns for their employees.

There appear to be no practical or theoretical grounds for claiming that screening of this type would be any more successful in older age groups, while its adoption on a large scale would certainly divert scarce resources and trained staff from more useful and beneficial activities.

Screening for Hypertension in Old Age

There has been so much argument and debate about treatment of hypertension in old age that a separate mention is necessary, together with guidance upon whether treatment is justified. Unfortunately, the whole area is unclear with rival camps expressing strong and often dogmatic views, despite the absence of convincing scientific evidence based upon careful controlled trials.

In this debate it is wise to remember the admonition by Oliver (1982) on the dangers in treating risk factors with drugs. He has pointed out that only a small minority of individuals with a given risk factor will actually develop the disease while, if all are given drug treatment, they are all then exposed to the risk of adverse reactions. The net result in some trials may be an actual increase in morbidity or even in mortality (e.g. the clofibrate trial in ischaemic heart disease resulted in a higher total mortality in the treated group as compared to the controls). Oliver added that 'aggressiveness in the use of these drugs should be inversely proportional to age' and this advice certainly applies to decisions on whether to employ hypotensive therapy.

It is now fairly clear that up to the age of 70 or 75 raised systolic, diastolic or mean blood pressure carries an increased risk of ischaemic heart disease and stroke and there is reasonable evidence, up to these ages, that careful hypotensive therapy for pressures above 160/90 will be of benefit to the patients. The recommended treatment is usually a thiazide diuretic and it is important to remember that the hypotensive effect of a small dose is as great as that of a larger dose although the risk of adverse reaction is greater with the latter. Hence 2·5 mg of bendrofluazide would be the recommended dose and if that did not produce satisfactory blood pressure levels, then a small dose of a beta-adrenergic blocking agent should be added, e.g. 50 mg daily of atenolol or metoprolol. At the present time much is being written about the usefulness of vasodilators (especially calcium antagonists and inhibitors of angiotensin-converting enzyme) as first-line treatment for hypertension. As far as we are aware, there is not yet enough information on their medium and long-term effects in old patients to justify their routine use in this age group.

What then ought to be our policy for the management of patients aged 75 or more who have raised blood pressure? The honest answer is that we do not at present have the knowledge on which to base rational treatment policies. In considering this problem, we have to question whether raised blood pressure has the same significance in an 80-year-old person as in someone who is young or middle-aged. The 80-year-old is likely to have a rather rigid and inelastic arterial tree and hence the systolic pressure may have to be higher in order to ensure delivery of a given volume of blood in a given time. Attempts to reduce blood pressure in these circumstances may therefore lead to reduced tissue perfusion. It is necessary to consider the possible effects upon cerebral blood flow of such a reduction. There are complex safeguards designed to protect the brain from under-perfusion resulting from decreases in blood pressure or cardiac output and even where there are dramatic reductions, cerebral blood flow is maintained at normal levels. As with other homeostatic mechanisms, there is often a reduction in efficiency in old age and this auto-regulation may frequently be significantly impaired. Hence meddle-some attempts at blood pressure reduction may seriously threaten cerebral blood flow and the decision to employ hypotensive therapy in persons over 75 must be taken with *extreme caution*.

Of course, where there is clinical evidence of ill effects from hypertension then reduction should be sought. Thus in a patient with high pressure and angina or evidence of left ventricular strain, then reduction is indicated, but even in these circumstances sudden and precipitate reductions must be avoided since serious consequences are likely.

Before deciding to treat, blood pressure should be repeatedly measured over a period of weeks or even months since initial levels are often misleadingly high. Where possible, pressures should be measured in the patient's own home where she is most likely to be relaxed and at ease. During the introduction of the hypotensive régime regular blood pressure checks should be made with the patient *supine and erect*. This should continue as long as the patient is on the hypotensive drug since postural hypotension may supervene at any stage.

Should general practitioners (or other primary team members) be screening elderly patients for hypertension? We find this an uncomfortable question to answer since we fear that ill-timed and over-enthusiastic screening and treatment (especially in the oldest age groups) could readily lead to serious side-effects. The fact that around three-quarters of old people have occasion to see their general practitioner at least once a year probably offers sufficient opportunity for blood pressure checks.

Finally, it is important to emphasize that vague unsteadiness of gait and complaints of giddiness, etc. are very common in old age (*see* Chapter 3) and if an 80-year-old female with such symptoms is found to have a blood pressure of 180/100, it is most improbable that lowering it to 150/90 will make her more stable and, indeed, if postural hypotension is thereby induced, her balance may be made much worse.

CASE FINDING

The process of case finding is fundamentally different from screening in that it is an attempt to discover actual symptomatic disease which is already affecting the patient and producing loss or disturbance of function.

It has already been pointed out in Chapter 1 that old people often do not behave rationally in relation to disability and may fail to seek appropriate help from their medical attendants. This phenomenon was studied in Edinburgh more than twenty years ago and the term 'non-reporting' was invented (Williamson *et al.* 1964). It was found that about half the conditions afflicting the old people who were studied had not been reported to their general practitioners. More detailed study indicated that these patients were selective in what they brought to medical notice.

Figure 8.1 shows the degree of non-reporting associated with conditions of heart, lungs and nervous system.

It will be seen that the general practitioner's awareness of these conditions was quite high. Presumably the old people had an expectation that their doctor would be able to improve these conditions and hence felt impelled to tell him about them. It is possible also that the doctor had signalled in some way that he was interested and available for help in these circumstances.

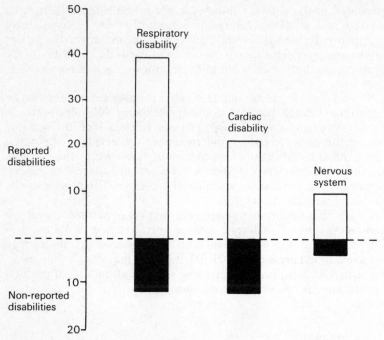

Fig. 8.1. The degree of non-reporting associated with disabilities of heart, lungs and nervous system.

By contrast the conditions shown in *Fig.* 8.2 were largely un-reported.

These poorly reported conditions include such conditions as chronic joint disease, many foot problems and abnormalities of bladder function (mostly prostatism in males and degrees of stress or urge incontinence in females). These were conditions which old people tended to consider not worth bringing to the attention of their practitioners, presumably believing there was little prospect of benefit thereby. Perhaps it was the fatalism of old age and the attitude that 'nothing could be done about it' since 'it is just old age'? There also exists the possibility that some doctors managed to convey an impression of low interest in these conditions and little optimism about their ability to help. No matter why these conditions remained unreported, they are important disabilities. Joint and foot conditions are unpleasant and painful and may rapidly lead to restricted movement which, in turn, may lead to reduction in pleasurable activities and in time interfere with important social activities. Eventually essential tasks such as self-care, shopping and catering may be impaired with

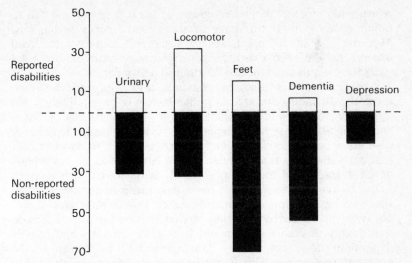

Fig. 8.2. The degree of non-reporting associated with urinary, locomotor and foot disabilities together with dementia and depression.

obvious dangers to health. Bladder disturbance is unpleasant and also may readily become a humiliation to the patient. All these conditions therefore may reduce self-esteem and morale which is already a danger in old age because of social and economic disadvantages. Equally disturbing was the high level of non-reported dementia although this is perhaps easier to understand since, even quite early in the dementing process, the patient is apt to lose insight into the nature of his/her predicament and thus is unlikely to make appropriate judgements and decisions as to what to do. It is perhaps more surprising that relatives or others had not sought help for these patients. The large proportion of unreported depression is also alarming since this is an extremely unpleasant experience for the patients and it is generally treatable, while if left untreated it carries the risk of serious secondary consequences such as malnutrition and social isolation or even death from suicide.

Recent claims have been made that this phenomenon of non-reporting is no longer a significant problem and that, since three-quarters of old people consult their general practitioner at least once a year, these general practitioners must be well aware of any serious problems. It is probable that this is partly true—indeed it would be surprising and very disappointing had no improvement occurred. The fact remains, however, that some disabilities still come to light only at an advanced stage. It must still be quite common for an old person to consult her doctor about her cough or breathlessness and fail to mention her painful stiff knee or troublesome corns or bunions. Moreover, as already pointed out in Chapter 2, there is widespread unawareness of the existence of cognitive impairment in older patients, even those in touch with medical personnel.

Arising from these findings, demands have been made for some form of case finding and several studies have now been published. No large controlled studies comparable to the South-east London Screening Study have been carried out so it is not possible to quantify benefits or cost effectiveness. Despite this, however, many will accept that early diagnosis is always better than late; indeed this is the basis of most traditional medical practice. It is obvious that it is much better to know that an old lady has osteoarthritis of her knees before she develops flexion contractures, since this disaster can almost always be prevented by quite simple rehabilitation measures. Likewise it is highly desirable that an old lady with dementia and heavily dependent upon her nearby daughter should be known to the appropriate services. This is not because we can do much for her dementia (although we may be able to avoid some of its secondary consequences), but because we must do everything we can to protect the daughter from exhaustion, frustration or demoralization so that she may feel able to continue her caring role.

From what has been said above, it will be clear that case finding in old age is a wide-ranging and complex process which involves the planned detection of established disability (including mental disability) as well as the detection of social and family precariousness. Hence the objective is not merely the diagnosis of disease in one or more organs, nor is it merely the assessment of the patient as an individual, rather it is the assessment of the patient as an integral part of a complex social unit which is usually the family but may in some cases involve non-family supporters such as friends or neighbours.

Who is to do the Case Finding?

Studies in Edinburgh by Buckley and Runciman (1985) have shed interesting light on this question. They made a short videorecord of an old lady at home talking to Miss Runciman. In the course of this, the old lady answered some questions, made several observations about being a burden to her family and rather painfully got out of her chair and moved about the room. This record was then shown to different groups including general practitioner trainees, established principals, students of physiotherapy, students of social work and student district nurses and health visitors. Each viewer was asked to write down all the problems which they identified during the recording. The results showed quite striking group differences with each group tending to see only the items relevant to their own interests while apparently not being aware of other significant problems. Thus the doctors tended to mention only that the patient had an arthritic hip and angina, the physiotherapy students noticed the patient's difficulty in rising from the chair, her slow gait and poor postural control. The students of social work actually appeared to have the best performance because not only did they mention the patient's medical and mobility problems but also indicated that she was worrying about her daughters and her own relationship with them. It almost seemed as though the extent of the observer's training was inversely related to the range of their observations or, in other words, all observers had some degree of tunnel vision but the medically trained person's tunnel was the narrowest.

This study has emboldened us to state our previously intuitively held opinion that the professional training and background of the case finder are much less important than his/her attitudes and degree of interest. The person who is interested in the old person's life style, hopes and fears and who understands the problems of guilt and anxiety which commonly afflict family carers is much more likely to get satisfaction from case finding and to make a success of it. Conversely, the doctor who has been programmed by his training to make a pathological diagnosis and to provide a specific remedy may be less interested in what may appear to be these more mundane and time-consuming considerations.

Generally, therefore, a nursing member of the primary care team will be selected for this task (or more often she will select herself). We do not believe that a doctor is usually suitable because much of the inquiry could appear irksome to him and he is perhaps 'too highly trained' for this task (or is this a euphemism for 'has too narrow a view'?).

Another important requirement for success in case finding is for the sharing and pooling of information about patients and families. Quite often the general practitioner will be in touch with an old patient who is also receiving help from the district nurse. It may be also that the health visitor is involved with another member of the family such as a daughter or daughter-in-law. We have inquired repeatedly among the general practitioners who attended our courses about the degree to which such information may be made available to other members of the primary team and we were surprised to learn that, even if they are all working from the same practice premises or health centre, it is quite unusual for even important data to be pooled or exchanged. This finding was also made by Buckley and Runciman.

This is obviously an unsatisfactory situation and yet it ought to be capable of being improved by simple and inexpensive means. The first requirement is that team members recognize the deficiency and are convinced that appropriate exchange of information is in their and the patients' interests. In geriatric medicine team members meet at least weekly for such purposes and although the situation is very different in general practice, some arrangement of this sort would at least provide a starting point and would certainly be better than failing to offer regular opportunities for team members to talk to each other in time set aside for this purpose. It is probable that, with the pressure on everyone's time, many may imagine that they cannot spare the time to indulge in such luxuries. Nothing could be further from the truth!

What should be the Scope of Case Finding?

Once more we have to rely on incomplete data since no one has successfully answered this question (indeed few have even posed it).

Despite this, however, certain principles may be proposed. The first is that the search should not be solely for disease but rather for loss of or disturbance in function. The second is that 'function' in this sense should be taken to include physical, mental and social function and, equally important, *family function*.

We have no doubt that the best place to make a complex assessment of this type is in the patient's home where she is more at ease and able to 'take on' the case finder on her own terms. The home environment can be assessed and, as will be shown, this may offer many clues to the patient's problems. Family members or neighbours, where involved, can demonstrate the sources of their anxiety such as dangerous stairs, evidence of poor housekeeping or inadequate food supplies in the house.

We have suggested that case finding by a nurse observer should involve two levels of inquiry:

(1) where the observer detects problems and acts upon them, and

(2) where the problems are referred to the general practitioner.

It is convenient to start with some sort of check list and we offer some suggestions for this (*Tables* 8.1 and 8.2), but it is to be hoped that each case finder will gradually evolve her own way of doing the investigation which suits her own particular methods of establishing rapport with old people.

Suggestions for a Check List

Table 8.1 comprises a list of items for observation and for acting upon.

This last particular part of case finding (*Family function*) may be very tricky as family members may have difficulty in expressing their feelings and may resent inquiries even if very tactfully carried out. The hard-pressed middle-aged woman trying to offer support to her ageing parent and simultaneously coping with her tasks as mother, wife, household manager and employee has been aptly described as 'the woman in the middle'.

Table 8.1. 'Observe and act' items

Social function
  (*a*) *Detection of expressed loneliness*
    Assessment of attitudes

    How often visited by $\left\{\begin{array}{l}\text{family members?} \\ \text{non-family members?} \\ \text{statutory or voluntary services?}\end{array}\right.$

    Membership of social   Church, club, lunch club, recreational activities
      organizations
    Patient's attitudes to   Satisfaction, resentment or guilt at amount of
      family   family support

  (*b*) *Home premises*
    Has there been recent rehousing (or other relocation)?
    General state of home—cleanliness, tidiness, malodorous
    Adequacy of heating/insulation in living room, bedroom and bathroom
    Diet and catering—food stores, food in refrigerator, means for cooking, number
      of pots/pans in regular use
    Evidence of alcohol or tobacco abuse

Physical function
  (*a*) *Mobility*
    How far can patient walk, can she manage stairs?
    Walking aids
    Inspect gait and footwear
  (*b*) *Postural stability*
    Observe patient rise from chair, walk across room, turn and return to chair
    Are bed, chair and toilet seat correct height?
    Where patient is unsteady, measure blood pressure, erect and supine

Mental function
    Mental status tests (*see* Chapter 2) of cognitive function
    State of house and patient's appearance
    Is patient currently managing shopping, pension, etc.?
    Detection of anxiety or mood disturbance (*see* Appendix at end of this chapter)

Family function
  (*a*) Identify the principal carer (usually daughter or daughter-in-law)
  (*b*) Interview principal carer separately
    Level of satisfaction with present circumstances?
  (*c*) Effect of caring for patient on her other roles (wife, mother, household
    manager and employee)
  (*d*) Fears, hopes and expectations for the future
    Present cost of care (travelling, time spent per week, etc.)

Not infrequently, even the chance to speak to someone who under-stands is a considerable relief to a daughter who is beginning to feel the strains of responsibility. An outline of potential help and support now and in the future often gives her the fortitude to continue her support for much longer.

Where there is evidence of stress, frustration, resentment or fatigue then there is urgent need for action since, if unrelieved, the carer may crack under the strain and this is usually irreversible. Yet we repeatedly find that general practitioners do not seem to appreciate this. Thus we have referrals in which the practitioner says: 'This old lady has been causing problems for months but knowing you are so short of beds I have tried to steer her away from you for as long as possible. Her daughter now seems to be at the end of her tether and is

Table 8.2. 'Observe and refer to general practitioner' items

(*a*) *Cardiorespiratory*
Cough, sputum, wheeze
Dyspnoea, orthopnoea, angina
Cyanosis, arrhythmia, oedema

(*b*) *Locomotor*
Difficulty in walking or transferring
Pain, stiffness, weakness, tremor
Examine gait and footwear

(*c*) *Bladder*
Frequency of micturition; nocturia; dysuria; incontinence; prostatism

Bowel
Pattern of bowel function; recent alteration in pattern or increase in laxative consumption

(*d*) *Postural disturbance*
History of falls or syncope
Unsteady gait
Postural hypotension
Hazards in home

(*e*) *Vision*
Simple assessment; read newsprint; examine spectacles

(*f*) *Hearing*
No obvious hearing problem noted
Occasional items had to be repeated
Voice had to be raised, frequent repetition
Great difficulty, having to shout, write messages, etc.

(*g*) *Medication*
Seek out prescribed and non-prescribed medicines
Does patient know what each is for and dosage regime?
Dates on containers

---

demanding that something must be done.' Nothing could be more mistaken than this attitude and usually where a daughter is genuinely 'at the end of her tether' this represents a failure of the system, usually a failure to understand the urgency of such need.

Table 8.2 comprises a relatively small list of items for observation and referral to the patient's general practitioner.

Who is to Receive Case Finding?

Some enthusiasts have suggested that everyone over 65 years of age should receive case finding. This is not only impracticable, but it would represent a huge waste of scarce resources and divert them from much more urgent activities.

We wish to propose some apparent danger groups. Some are self-evidently high risk while others may be only marginally so.

The undoubted danger groups are:

1. The widowed, especially where widowhood has been preceded by a long period of caring for a disabled and dependent spouse. Where there is an absence of caring and supportive relatives, the danger is increased.
2. Those with known chronic disabling conditions such as arthropathy, stroke, parkinsonism, etc. Also those known to be dementing or with history of depression.
3. Those recently discharged from hospital, especially the strangely misclassified 'social admissions'.
4. Those already recognized as having special needs, e.g. already receiving home help or meals-on-wheels.
5. The very old (85+) living alone or with an equally aged spouse. Four-fifths of this age group need help with basic living activities.
6. Those recently relocated, e.g. where an old person has moved house; especially if the removal was not an elective but an enforced procedure, as when an old area is demolished and the old person rehoused in a new estate.

Other high-risk groups should be identified in the light of peculiarly stressful local conditions, e.g. old people living in certain areas of multiple deprivation may become fearful of vandalism or the activities of disaffected youngsters.

Some have suggested that certain categories of patients on repeat prescriptions should be under special surveillance, e.g. those on diuretics, hypoglycaemic drugs and psychotropics.

In recent years it has been suggested that it is possible to identify those with significant unmet needs by sending a postal questionnaire to patients over 65 on practice lists. Barber *et al.* (1980) devised a nine-point questionnaire which they showed was capable of accurate selection of patients with unmet needs. This has the considerable disadvantage that 80 per cent of respondents answered the questionnaire in such a way that they had to be visited by a practice nurse, thus only saving 20 per cent of visits in a fully comprehensive case-finding scheme. Further refinements have succeeded in making the questionnaire more discriminating and promising results have recently come from the United States. One useful instrument is the Duke University 5-item screener (Duke OARS, 1978). This contains the following questions:

1. Can you get to places which are out of walking distance?
2. Can you go shopping?
3. Can you prepare your own meals?
4. Can you do your housework?
5. Can you handle your own money?

Future research may indicate that the use of a 'screening instrument' such as the above will accurately and cheaply pinpoint those old persons with important unmet needs, who may then be subjected to assessment along the lines indicated in this chapter.

SUMMARY AND CONCLUSION

Despite the evidence of the ineffectiveness of multiphasic screening and the absence of convincing proof of the benefits of case finding, we believe that, even today, too many old people and their carers only come to medical notice when the situation is approaching the dimensions of a crisis.

Although there have been improvements over the past few decades, non-reporting of disability and loss of function is still a problem and systematic efforts at case finding should be devised by progressive primary care teams.

The case-finding process should be carried out by a nurse member of the team and should be directed at the detection of loss of function rather than disease processes. The functions to be assessed are physical, mental, social and family.

It is necessary to decide which groups of old people are at special risk and to concentrate the case finding upon them. Some groups are obviously in danger, e.g. those with chronic physical or mental disability, while others may be in danger because of purely local circumstances. Postal questionnaires have been shown to be capable of identifying vulnerable old people.

Evidence is now accumulating that case finding reduces future hospital inpatient stay and that the general well-being and morale of old persons are improved (by comparison with controls). We feel that participation in this kind of activity may have an indirect benefit by raising the interest of the team members who are involved. Anything which enhances interest in older patients must be beneficial in helping to counteract the prevailing negative attitudes towards old age.

APPENDIX

ASSESSMENT OF MENTAL STATUS

Cognitive function should be assessed along the lines outlined in Chapter 2 using the 'set test' and the Isaacs–Walkey test (or local equivalents).

The condition of the house and the patient's appearance will be taken into account and inquiries will be made as to the patient's ability to manage her finances, her shopping, paying rent and fuel bills, etc.

Detection of Anxiety and Mood Disturbance

This may be simple or extremely difficult depending on the manner in which the disturbance presents. We would like to suggest a series of questions which have been used in an elderly Scottish population and which have proved to be acceptable and discriminating. We have not attempted to attribute special significance to any of these questions and they are to be regarded rather as the sort of inquiry which will enable the observer to uncover mood disturbance in the patient.

The patient's speed of response should be noted as: notably quick, normal speed, slower than average or retarded. The patient's attitude should also be noted, whether agitated and restless or withdrawn and avoiding eye-to-eye contact.

The suggested questions are as follows:

1. Have you any anxieties or problems which worry you at present?
   If yes: (*a*) Are you feeling upset by this?
          (*b*) Is there any other particular worry bothering you at present?
2. (*a*) Are there times when you feel anxious without really knowing why?
   (*b*) Are you distressed by silly pointless thoughts that keep coming into your mind against your will?
3. Have you any fears that tend to haunt or worry you?

The above three questions will uncover anxiety and the following are directed at the detection of mood disturbance:

4. What interests have you?
   If none: Have you lost interest in almost everything?
5. Do you look forward to things?
   If not or doubtful: Does the future seem pointless?
6. Do you find it a bother to do the things you are able to do?
   If yes: (a) Does even the thought of having to do anything feel an
             effort to you?
          (b) Do you sometimes have to push yourself to start even the
             simplest task?
7. Question to females: Do you tend to cry more often than you used to?
   Question to males: Have you felt like crying more recently than in the
             past?
8. (a) How are you in your spirits today?
       Are you happy or do you feel down?
   (b) Have your spirits been good or poor lately?
   (c) Have your spirits ever been so low that you have just sat for hours
       on end?
9. (a) How are you sleeping now?
   (b) Do you feel rested when you rise in the morning?
   (c) Has your sleep been good or poor in the past 12 months?
10. Do you sleep with or without sleeping tablets?
11. Have you felt nervous or depressed in the past 12 months?
    If yes: Do you feel better or worse now compared to then? Were you
             able to cope adequately with your everyday life when you felt
             like this?
12. Are you taking any medicines, tablets or capsules to soothe your nerves
    or make you less depressed?
    If yes: Do you know what you are taking?
13. (a) Do you enjoy your food?
    (b) Has your appetite been good or bad lately?
14. Would you say that you are content with your present way of life?
    Do you have any doubts about this?
    Are you dissatisfied?

Questions (4) to (14) may appear rather formidable to direct at an old person in the course of case finding, but this approach using these questions has been successfully used in Scotland and, provided the observer has already established some rapport with the patient, they have proved entirely acceptable. Each observer may wish to modify the questions a little to suit individual preferences. If all responses are negative, then there is no significant anxiety or mood disturbance. On the other hand, positive responses to questions (4), (5), (6) and (8) would be highly suggestive of depression, which would be amply confirmed by positive responses to any of the subsequent questions.

(We are most indebted to Dr Margaret Maule who devised and validated this questionnaire: Milne *et al.* 1972.)

ADDENDUM

The report of the European Working Party on Hypertension in the Elderly has been published since the foregoing was written (Amery et al., 1986).

Hypotensive therapy appeared to be of benefit for those aged 60–75 years, but no benefit was derived by those aged 80 years or more, which reinforces our message on page 144.

REFERENCES

Amery A., Birkenhager W., Brixko R. *et al.* (1986) Efficacy of antihypertensive drug treatment according to age, sex, blood pressure and previous cardiovascular disease in patients over the age of 60. *Lancet* **2**, 589.

Barber J. H., Willis J. B. and McKeating E. (1980) A postal screening questionnaire in preventive geriatric care. *J. R. Coll. Gen. Pract.* **30**, 49.

Buckley E. G. and Runciman P. J. (1985) Health assessment of the elderly at home. University of Edinburgh, Internal report.

Duke OARS (1978) *Multidimensional Functional Assessment: The OARS Methodology*, 2nd ed. Durham, N.C.: Duke University Medical Center.

Department of Health and Social Security (1976) *Prevention and Health: Everybody's Business.* London: HMSO.

Milne J. S., Maule M. M., Cormack S. *et al.* (1972) The design and testing of a questionnaire and examination to assess physical and mental health in older people using a staff nurse as the observer. *J. Chron. Dis.* **25**, 385.

Oliver M. F. (1982) Risks of correcting the risk of coronary disease and stroke with drugs. *New Eng. J. Med.* **306**, 297.

South-east London Screening Study Group (1977) A Controlled Trial of Multiphasic Screening in Middle-age. Results of the South-east London Screening Study. *Int. J. Epid.* **6**, 357.

Williamson J., Stokoe I. H., Gray S. *et al.* (1964) Old people at home: their unreported needs. *Lancet* **1**, 1117–20.

9 SERVICES FOR THE ELDERLY— HOW AND WHEN TO USE THEM

Previous chapters have emphasized the precariousness of some elderly people and the stresses upon their families. The complexity of these problems has been described and attention called to the inter-woven effects of age, disease and environmental factors.

Primary care team members may readily feel perplexed or even daunted by these matters and even more so by the bewildering array of services both statutory and voluntary. Further frustration may arise when difficulty is encountered in finding the correct portal of entry to a service which has been identified as appropriate for an individual patient. Frustration may change to anger if agencies then appear to surround themselves with barriers and indulge in the bureaucratic pastime of 'passing the buck'.

The past two decades have seen considerable increase in interest in services to the elderly by health and local authorities and politicians have responded to some extent to public unease at the inadequacy of some provisions. There has been much talk of the importance of community care and there have been declared policies of switching resources from institutional and 'acute' services to community and 'long-term' services. While this has only had limited results, there is no doubt that some services have been greatly improved, e.g. the home help service.

The effect has been rather patchy, however, with some areas of the country responding more enthusiastically than others to the demand for improved community care.

Some services are provided at national level, e.g. pensions and DHSS allowances, some are provided by local authorities, e.g. home helps and meals-on-wheels, and others are the responsibility of health authorities (general practitioner and community nursing services, hospital and specialist services). Others are provided by voluntary agencies such as the Red Cross and Women's Royal Voluntary Service.

As emphasized in Chapter 1, effective use of resources is based upon identification of patients' and carers' needs, followed by the

prompt supply of the appropriate service. This is frequently a complicated matter and often requires the skills of the geriatric multidisciplinary team.

Effective use of resources is dependent upon several factors: the
availability in adequate supply of resources, good communication
between all concerned, the mutual recognition of and respect for
each others' skills and professionalism. This should lead to a blurring
of role demarcations and a willingness among workers to share
information and participate in management decisions with the aim of
securing good coordination of activities and evaluation of jointly
agreed plans.

This chapter outlines the main services with which primary teams
should be familiar. An attempt has been made to emphasize how,
when and for whom these services should be sought. Some suggestions
are made as to possible beneficial organizational changes.

THE PRIMARY CARE TEAM

This is generally taken to mean the general practitioner, the district
nurse and the health visitor, but other members may have important
roles in certain settings, e.g. the practice manager (in larger practices)
and the secretary/receptionist in smaller firms. The effectiveness of
teamwork is dependent upon the interests of team members, their
personalities and the quality of management and organization. It is
obvious that where all share the same premises, teamwork is made
easier, but it is perfectly possible for doctors and nurses to have their
offices and consulting rooms next to each other and yet fail to work in
a proper team fashion, thereby losing the opportunity to pool their
skills and efforts for the maximum benefit of patients.

The General Practitioner

Many services for old people are not within the gift of the practitioner,
but despite this he tends to be widely regarded as the pivotal figure in
determining that the needs of patients are appropriately met. Most
old people and their families see him as the gatekeeper to services
which they feel they may need and expect him to have expert knowledge of all resources and be their advocate in seeing that their needs
are met expeditiously. This places great responsibility upon general
practitioners both in seeing that individual patient's needs are met
and in making sure that scarce resources are not squandered upon
those who do not genuinely need them.

Other professionals—social workers, housing managers and home help supervisors, for instance—may apply different criteria and have different priorities for the deployment of their services and this can lead to conflict and disagreement. It is important, therefore, that when making a referral to other agencies, full and accurate information should be given and, while it is reasonable to indicate what the general practitioner, the patient and others may expect from a service, it is not appropriate or helpful to 'promise' something that others may think is not necessary. The practitioner should bear in mind that other professionals, having made their own assessment of need, may justifiably reach a different conclusion and see a different service requirement from that which he has made. Thus it is much more tactful and polite to ask the geriatrician for help, rather than to demand admission or day-hospital care, just as it is better to ask a social worker for her opinion rather than to seek only residential accommodation.

Problems and misunderstandings persist and there are several fairly obvious reasons:

1. Quite often general practitioners have received little or no training in the availability and usefulness of services and may have erroneous notions on the roles of, for example, home help supervisors or wardens in sheltered housing. Thompson (1984) has pointed out that such knowledge is 'as important as is our knowledge of anatomy'.
2. The needs of old people and their families tend to be multiple and complex, as emphasized previously in this book, and their precise identification may be difficult; a simple pathological diagnosis is rarely a complete answer.
3. Services are themselves complex and this is made worse by the fact that the divisions and barriers between them were created in conditions which may have long since altered. For example, the two systems of long-term institutional care—that provided by the hospital service (for which there is no charge or means test) and that provided by local authorities (for which there is strict means testing and residents may have to pay the full cost)—no longer fulfil separate and clearly defined functions. Indeed, several studies have shown that residents in both these long-term sectors are remarkably similar, most being dependent, many confused and some incontinent. In urban areas there may be infuriating and unnecessary obstacles to efficiency such as when geriatric and psychogeriatric services do not have the same geographical boundaries to their catchment areas which, moreover, may not correspond with social work boundaries.

Often these deficiencies may be traced to no better reason than that the individuals concerned resist changes.

4. Another problem is that local provision may vary greatly. Thus the geriatric service in one area may provide a rapid response to requests for help with immediate admission to wards or day hospital, while an adjoining service is slow, defensive and evasive, sheltering behind lengthy waiting lists and lamentations about shortage of beds. Different voluntary and local authority residential homes may apply widely differing criteria for acceptability of old people for admission, varying from freely mobile and near-independent to severely dependent, demented with frequent incontinence. The present picture is even more unclear because of the current mushroom growth in private nursing homes with beds available for old people on DHSS supplementation.

The general practitioner is in the position of having the most complete view of the needs of old people in the community and also of the strengths and weaknesses of services. He should therefore be prepared to identify weaknesses and inefficiencies, whether in statutory or voluntary services, and to campaign both individually and collectively to secure improvements.

The District Nursing Service

The district nursing sister (or charge nurse for males) is a registered general nurse who has had a course of post-basic training and is responsible for providing skilled nursing care to patients in the community, including those in their own homes, in residential homes and in practice premises or health centres. Enrolled nurses and nursing auxiliaries may work under her direction to provide nursing care of a less skilled nature. This service provides 365-day cover and is available to all age groups (but 80 per cent of visits, both new and follow-up, are to patients aged 65 or more). A large majority of district nurses are 'practice attached' in the Edinburgh area. About 70 per cent are attached to general practices and medical centres and another 10 per cent are health centre based, while only 20 per cent are 'geographical', i.e. serve patients in a defined geographical area who may be looked after by many general practitioners from different practices. The policy of encouraging practice attachments helps to facilitate good teamwork, but it certainly does not guarantee it, just as 'geographical' disposition of nurses does not make it impossible.

The training of district nurses today recognizes that their work is mainly with the elderly and that more frail and dependent old people now remain in the community for much longer than previously. Much of the home nursing of old people consists of simple care such as washing, bathing, dressing and undressing. Where sufficient family support is available, these responsibilities will be met within family resources and home helps also are often involved (sometimes 'on the side'). Where circumstances dictate that this simple care falls to the district nursing service, this may result in considerable burdens with a commitment for up to 365 days each year to the patients concerned. The patient may require help several times a day and sometimes also at night and experiments have been conducted both here and abroad in providing such care as a means of avoiding hospital admission. This necessitates a considerable increase in district nurse personnel but not a large increase in fully trained staff. Much of the 'hands on' care can be provided by nursing auxiliaries with district nurse supervision. Variations of this provision have used home helps, while one French experiment invented a 'new carer' with a role encompassing those of home helps and nursing auxiliaries.

One frequent need is for someone to help the patient to rise and get dressed in the morning and to go to bed at night (as in patients with stroke or arthritic disabilities). It is generally fairly easy to cope with the morning tasks but only rarely can the service provide a 'putter-to-bed service', although this may be all that is required to keep the patient happily at home.

However the nursing service is organized and staffed, it is inevitable that the general practitioner will be providing all or most of the medical care, and success or failure may to a large extent depend upon the effectiveness of communication and teamwork.

In Chapter 8 we have suggested that a nurse member of the primary team should generally fill the role of case finder and often the district nurse will be the most suitable choice. However, she is often so hard-pressed and faces increasing demands from what seems to be an endless open-ended commitment that she may be forced to adopt defensive tactics. This sometimes results in the nurse taking a role as a performer of procedures rather than as a nurse looking after a patient. This is illustrated by the case of the nurse who attends an old lady to dress her leg ulcers. Over several months the old lady's condition deteriorates, she becomes immobile and there are incontinence problems. The nurse continues to visit regularly and perform the dressings but apparently remains unaware of the deterioration in function. Perhaps she has genuinely failed to notice, but it is much more likely that she preferred 'not to see', and consciously or subconsciously rejected the evidence of her own senses either because she would not have known what to do or because she felt certain that it would involve her in much more work with which she felt she could not cope. This anecdote is not an exaggeration, nor is it a criticism of the nurse; rather it indicates a common deficiency in primary care which is to respond to demand rather than need. It is the antithesis of case finding and underlines the need for an emphasis upon 'thinking preventively', genuine team effort and regular opportunities for exchange of information, plus good liaison with other services such as geriatric medicine.

An encouraging development in recent years has been the emergence of nurses with a special interest in continence. They are able to assess bladder function, identify factors involved in loss of continence and offer advice on management, including the supply of special clothing, appliances and equipment. These nurses work closely with geriatricians and understand the criteria for seeking full urodynamic investigations as outlined in Chapter 5. Practice nurses should be free to seek help from the continence nursing adviser either about individual patients or about problems in general. She thus fulfils two important functions—helping with individual patients and educating other district nurses (who, in turn, educate other team members).

Analogous roles are played by stoma-care nurses for patients with ileostomy or colostomy.

The Health Visitor

The health visitor is a general nurse who has completed a course of training in prevention and health education. She differs from most other nurses in that she has direct access to patients (and families) without waiting for them to be referred to her. She has a statutory obligation to visit certain categories of patients but these are all to do with maternity and child care.

The health visiting service was originally created in the late nineteenth century as a means of assuaging public alarm at the very high level of infant and child morbidity and mortality. The work of health visitors in antenatal and maternity care and in education of mothers in child rearing led to dramatic improvements in this sphere. Over the past few decades their range of activities has increased and they are now involved in mental health, diabetes and communicable and sexually transmitted diseases.

For several decades there has been speculation that health visitors should become more involved in the care of older patients, but the majority continue to be mainly interested in the problems at the other end of life. This is shown by the fact that only 10–20 per cent of patients visited by health visitors in Lothian were aged 65 or more (in contrast to 80 per cent of patients attended by district nurses). It therefore seems probable that, with some notable exceptions, the present generation of health visitors do not seek much greater involvement with the elderly.

We have already pointed out in Chapter 8 that the health visitor is, in theory, the ideal person to undertake case finding on account of her special training in prevention and health education, but we also argued that attitude, interest and enthusiasm are more relevant than formal training. Thus where a practice health visitor shows active interest, she should be encouraged to do case finding. Where this is not the case, a district nurse can readily fulfil this role.

Some geriatric and psychogeriatric services have specialist health visitors who act as liaison workers between the hospital (including day hospital) and community services. They help to ensure continuity of care especially for the period of special vulnerability when a patient has been discharged from hospital. It is important that this liaison should not be seen as a one-way flow of information from hospital to community, since it is equally important that knowledge of patients and families held by community nurses should be passed on to the hospital team. It is important that a health visitor attached to a hospital unit should not inadvertently lead to less communication between hospital nurses directly in contact with patients and 'hands on' nurses dealing with the same patients in the community. This could happen if the nurses concerned simply adopt the attitude of 'Leave it all to the liaison health visitor' instead of making attempts to establish direct personal contacts.

OTHER COMMUNITY HEALTH SERVICES

Many old people have relatively little contact with primary care, while having regular involvement with other community health services such as dentistry, optometry, chiropody and audiology. Younger and fitter old people nowadays can usually find out how to obtain these services, and certainly do so more successfully than twenty years ago. For the frailer old people, however, especially the housebound, access to these services often poses considerable problems. Not all dentists and opticians, for example, are specially interested in very old patients and only a few will undertake domiciliary treatment.

The *chiropody service* in the NHS is notoriously overstretched; patients in some areas have to wait up to 6 months for domiciliary treatment. This is a very long time to wait for relief from painful corns and calluses which may cause serious restrictions in mobility with the secondary consequences mentioned in Chapter 4. Some old people require only a nail-cutting service because they cannot reach their feet or cannot see well enough to cut their own nails safely. In some areas, therefore, a simple nail-cutting service is provided, but this leads to misgivings in case serious ischaemia is not recognized and tissue damage ensues with potentially disastrous results. General practitioners, district nurses and health visitors all have responsibility for identifying patients who need special help with feet care, and perhaps the general practitioner is the appropriate person to decide whether nail cutting may be done by someone other than a trained chiropodist. Old people (and relatives on their behalf) may make direct requests for help to the chiropody service.

Other community services include *domiciliary physiotherapy* which has proved very valuable in selected cases. Its main use is in restoring mobility (and confidence) after relatively minor injury or after an intercurrent illness. It is especially valuable where the patient was already frail and perhaps showing some evidence of dementia. In these cases removal to a hospital ward or day hospital may be upsetting and benefits may be outweighed by disadvantages. Physiotherapy in these circumstances may be most appropriately provided in the patient's home. We emphasize that this provision cannot succeed where the need is for extensive rehabilitation as after a major stroke or more serious injury, in which the patient will require at least an initial period of rehabilitation in hospital or day hospital. Rehabilitation in these cases is not just a matter of 30 minutes daily from the physiotherapist, but extends through the whole 24 hours (in inpatients) or 5–6 hours (in day-hospital cases) being provided by occupational therapists and, most important, since present all the time, nursing staff. An example of inappropriate use of the domiciliary physiotherapy service was the case of the frail old lady in a residential home. She had previously had a stroke with right hemiparesis and had been rehabilitated to independent mobility as an inpatient in the geriatric unit about two years previously. She had been appropriately placed in residential care on the death of her sister with whom she had lived and had managed well with minor help from staff with dressing and toileting. In April she developed a moderately severe chest infection and was laid up for 10 days after which she could not walk. The community physiotherapy service was summoned and visited her two or three times per week for 20–30 minutes. Little else seemed to have happened presumably because she was 'getting physiotherapy'. In August she was referred to the geriatric service but by this time she had a flexion contracture of the right knee. Despite admission and strenuous efforts on everyone's part (including the patient), she never walked again. This was an example of failure to realize the complexity of a patient's rehabilitation needs and that from the time of her chest infection she needed the skills of the full geriatric team.

Another useful service is the *laundry service* now offered in some areas to patients and families coping with incontinence. This and the continence nursing adviser have already been described in Chapter 5.

The adequacy or otherwise of these services listed above varies considerably from area to area or even from one part of a city to another. General practitioners have a duty to identify deficiencies and inefficiencies and to draw them to the attention of the responsible authorities. Beyond that, they, like other health professionals, have an obligation to inform their patients if they are not receiving the services which are supposed to be available in the Health Service.

SOCIAL SERVICES

Services Provided by Central Government

Some social services are provided by the Department of Health and Social Services, e.g. *supplementary allowances* for those with special needs and limited means. The whole field of welfare benefits is extremely complicated; even DHSS officials who operate the system admit to frustration and perplexity from time to time. Studies on uptake of allowances by older people, which have been carried out in several areas, have shown that this group does not receive all the benefit to which it is entitled. This is thought to be due to several factors: a lack of understanding of 'the system' by old people and those around them, poor advice from professionals, including social workers and doctors (which is due, in turn, to ignorance), and an innate abhorrence of asking for, and receiving, 'charity'.

Professional groups working with old people, and in a position to advise and influence them, should be aware of the major benefits to which they may be entitled. Local DHSS offices are prepared (and, in our experience, more than willing) to discuss benefit issues with the individual concerned. Pension books contain a slip which can be sent to the local DHSS office to request such a meeting. The national voluntary organization, Age Concern, produces a useful booklet each year—*Your Rights*—which explains the major financial issues for old people. Whilst it is written for old people themselves, it provides a valuable reference document for the consulting room.

One particular allowance deserves further mention here. The *attendance allowance* can be paid to disabled and dependent people of any age, and it is not means tested. There are two levels of payment: the lower for people who require help during either the day or night, and the higher for those who need 'round-the-clock' assistance. When a disabled person or his/her relative applies for the attendance allowance, he/she will be visited and assessed by an independent doctor. Many applications are turned down because the old person and/or the carer is not able to give a clear account of his/her level of dependency. In a significant proportion of these cases, the unsuccessful applications which go forward to appeal have the initial decision reversed. The general practitioner has a key role, both in advising people to apply for attendance allowance in the first instance, and in ensuring that they know how to put their case in the most effective way.

The amount of money involved is not large, but may allow the dependent person to afford enough extra help to enable him/her to stay at home, and to relieve stress on the main carer. If the latter has given up his or her job to do the caring and is below pensionable age, he or she is eligible for the *invalid care allowance*.

Expert advice on eligibility and method of application may be available in many districts from organizations such as the Disablement Income Group or the Citizens' Advice Bureau.

Other centrally funded services are *heating allowances* for help in meeting the costs of heating during times of severe cold. These appear to operate erratically and variably from area to area.

Recently *DHSS supplements* have become available for old people to enter private nursing or residential homes. This has stimulated a very rapid expansion in this form of provision, which has led to misgivings that some old people may be deprived of their independence by being persuaded to go into care unnecessarily. There are also worries lest the standard of care may not be good enough in some homes where the levels of trained staff are low.

We shall not discuss the matter of *income* in old age except to emphasize that it should be sufficient to enable pensioners to lead full and independent lives without fear of poverty or deprivation. In this respect, the UK does not compare at all well with many other European countries where state pensions may be as much as 60–70 per cent of average earnings. The present generation of old people contains many who have lived fairly meagre lives in the lean years between the wars and whose expectations are low. Future generations may not be so easily satisfied.

Local Authority Social Services
Local authorities are responsible for a wide range of services, many of them of the greatest importance to older people.

The existence of services which are separately funded, staffed and managed by health and social services can be a source of waste and inefficiency. This may be due to gaps between the services, e.g. in many areas there are problems over the provision of institutional care for old people with dementia severe enough to prevent them from living in the community, but without need for psychiatric care. Such patients may fall between two stools with both health and social services claiming that it is the other's responsibility. Some local authorities in England and Wales have responded by providing special homes (Elderly Mentally Infirm or 'EMI' Homes), but this has not been widely adopted, and in Scotland there have been two reports on the matter, one saying it was a local authority responsibility, the other that it was up to the Health Service. Predictably the result has been stalemate and serious misplacement of this 'unpopular' group of patients in acute wards (general medicine and orthopaedic surgery), in geriatric wards and in ordinary residential homes, where they may cause great problems by wandering, etc.

Other sources of inefficiency relate to overlapping of services where social and health resources are used for similar or identical purposes. Another serious problem may arise when a patient needs to move from one system to another and thereby has to overcome bureaucratic barriers, e.g. when a patient in hospital improves to the extent that she no longer needs hospital care but cannot go home, there may be delays and prevarications about arranging her transfer to residential accommodation. Another anomaly already referred to is that in hospital there is no charge for patients (although, after 13 weeks, the state pension is reduced), whereas in residential homes there is strict means testing and residents may have to pay the full economic cost from the day of admission. In these circumstances, it is not surprising that old people (and their relatives who hope to inherit) often prefer old people to remain as long as possible within the hospital sector.

In England and Wales there is a statutory obligation for health and local authorities to work together through joint consultative committees. Despite earnest attempts, however, effective joint planning and delivery of services are often ineffective and this is not surprising since both authorities are short of resources, face increasing demands and therefore may be reluctant to adopt jointly agreed plans which so often require additional monies.

SOCIAL WORKERS

Social workers are usually generic, i.e. they work with all client groups and do not concentrate specially upon such groups as older people. In this respect they are akin to general practitioners. While general practitioners are primarily concerned with diagnosis and treatment of disease, social workers are more involved in identifying the strengths and weaknesses of patients and their supporters. Some general practitioners will maintain that they too now adopt this wider approach and may add that social workers could usefully adopt some lessons from primary care. Thus a busy general practitioner will find it very frustrating to be told that resources needed for his patient are in short supply and that it may take days or weeks even to arrange a visit from the social worker.

The result may be that general practitioners and, to a lesser extent, community nurses may misunderstand the social worker's value and may even become mistrustful. Doctors and nurses have usually learned to get along together since they share bonds of tradition and training and operate within the familiar framework of the 'medical model' of diagnosis and treatment. Recently with cuts in local authority finances, services which were barely coping are now obviously seriously inadequate. This, together with the understandable preoccupation of social workers with the appalling problems of child abuse, has often meant that the availability of trained social workers for the elderly has been reduced to pitiful levels, leading to delays in provision and further disenchantment on the part of doctors and nurses.

This is all most unfortunate, since the help of an interested social worker may be extremely useful to the primary care team. It is wrong to regard the modern social worker as little more than the reincarnation of the 'lady almoner' of previous years, whose task was to be a provider of welfare or to arrange admission to an institution. A good social worker is expert at investigating sources of family dissension or strife and at identifying and reinforcing family strengths and resources. In this context, we are generally content to entrust to our social worker colleague most of the arrangements for respite care, since she is usually in the best position to monitor levels of family stress and recognize when the head of steam is approaching a level at which the safety valve of respite admission is indicated.

The Domiciliary Occupational Therapist

This community worker, based in the social services department, is often of great assistance to old people and their families by teaching them how best to cope with circumstances in the home. This is achieved first by skilled assessment of the nature of the disability, by measures aimed at restoration of lost function and lastly, where permanent disability exists, the supply of aids and equipment to compensate for the deficits. Often the instruction of carers on how to manage the patient is just as important as work with the individual patient. Thus it is equally as important to tell relatives what not to do as what to do. They must be instructed never to do things for patients which they can do for themselves, otherwise this ability may be rapidly and permanently lost. The occupational therapist is mainly concerned with competence in daily living: dressing, washing, toileting, moving safely and freely about the house, managing on and off bed, chair and toilet, skills in cooking and making light snacks, etc. The provision of aids and appliances, while important and 'visible', may often be of less importance than detailed assessment and education of patients and supporters.

The domiciliary occupational therapist ought to work closely with the team from the geriatric unit, and it is good practice for patient, domiciliary occupational therapist and hospital occupational therapist to meet in the patient's home as a means towards the planning of optimum arrangements for the patient's return home. A representative from primary care may usefully participate in such a predischarge home visit, usually the district nurse. It is possible to suggest others who might join in this activity, but there is a danger then that the occasion may readily become something of an invasion!

We strongly recommend that members of the primary team should become personally acquainted with their occupational therapy colleagues, both in the geriatric unit and the community. They certainly have much common ground and things to learn from and teach each other.

The Home Help Service

We believe that a well-run home help service is the lynch pin of community care for the elderly and may well be the 'jewel in the crown' of the British system. Characteristically its excellence is often unrecognized and almost always unsung. We never fail to be impressed by the effectiveness, skill and versatility of home helps and their supervisors.

It is perhaps of interest to record a little of the history of this service and some may be surprised to learn that it had its origins as a simple domestic support service for mothers recovering after childbirth. In those early days only basic domestic support was needed without special skills since household and family management remained firmly in the hands of the mother as mater familias. Recruitment to the service in those early days was often difficult both because it was an era of 'full employment' and because the job was generally regarded as being of low esteem and lacking job satisfaction. Now the situation has changed completely; 95 per cent of persons who receive the service are old and individual home helps daily receive confirmation of the important role they perform in making the lives of their clients tolerable, and even enjoyable.

With the recognition of the importance of this service there has been another important development: the appearance of expert home help supervisors whose management task has been to assess patients' needs and match these by the selection of home helps with the required attributes and qualities. This has resulted in great improvements in efficiency since each case is individually monitored so that the service's contribution may be increased, decreased or ceased as needs change.

Home helps are ostensibly untrained, but most are females approaching or at middle age who have considerable practical experience in household management and are competent in family and 'person' management. Most are or have been married, have reared families and have experience of elderly relatives. They have learned how to cope with families, husbands and households, often on very meagre budgets and to state that they are untrained is often a travesty of the truth. Their lack of formal training may be an asset since it enables them to establish relationships with their clients which is quite different (and generally more 'normal') than relationships with more formally trained staff such as doctors, nurses and therapists. We have often been enormously impressed by the subtly instinctive way in which a home help provides substantial help to an aged woman while preserving the notion (often an illusion) that she remains in complete control of her domain. This is in marked contrast to the 'professional' who inevitably tends to 'take over' and manage the situation in line with professional expectations.

In the UK, home helps manage to maintain large numbers of old people in their own homes who, in other circumstances (and in other parts of the world), would be in institutions. A substantial reduction in home helps would immediately result in disruption of hospital services for all adults. The list of duties which are required of home helps is lengthy, yet many certainly undertake tasks well beyond their call of duty simply because they are decent, caring persons who respond to the needs of the old people entrusted to their care. Their customary responsibilities such as shopping, collecting prescriptions and paying bills all place home helps in positions of trust. They also commonly help old people to get dressed and undressed, help them with toileting and grooming and in other intimate personal tasks. Although many authorities indicate that home helps should not assume responsibility for supervision of medication, many are involved in the laying out, day by day, of their elderly charges' tablets.

Home help supervisors become valuable repositories of information about old people with whom they are involved. There are powerful arguments in favour of primary care personnel getting to know their home help supervisors and establishing cordial relationships.

Home helps are paid an hourly rate for the job and patients in receipt of this service may be required to contribute towards this cost. Occasionally patients who would greatly benefit from a home help may display reluctance through unwillingness to make this contribution and this may lead to problems. In some areas it has been shown that the cost of means testing and levying charges exceeds the revenue thus realized. Is there scope for rationalization here?

Meals-on-Wheels

The meals-on-wheels service is usually run as a joint enterprise between the social services and a voluntary organization such as the Women's Royal Voluntary Service. Meals are prepared either commercially or in a local authority kitchen (as, for example, in a residential home) and delivered in heated containers by volunteers. Recipients of meals make a small contribution to the cost of the service. The service is excellent for old people who have a relatively short-term need, e.g. when there is a period of increased dependency during and for a few weeks after an illness. It is less satisfactory for long-term need as the ideal arrangement is to provide company with the meal since eating is a fundamentally important social occasion. Many old people will eat well if joined by friends or relatives but just pick at food if left on their own. In these circumstances enrolment in a lunch club or day centre should be sought wherever possible.

Day Centres and Lunch Clubs

This heading covers a wide range of facilities: from small lunch clubs, which meet once a week in a church hall and rely on volunteers to bring the old people and prepare the meals, to large, purpose-built day centres, open 5 days a week, with paid staff and a couple of tail-lift buses. At one end of the spectrum, the local community may try to meet a need which it has identified itself, without recourse to statutory funds. At the other end, the social work department may organize and fund a centre without using voluntary help at all. Most day centres and lunch clubs fall between these extremes and demonstrate the way in which a statutory body can work closely with voluntary organizations.

Ten to fifteen years ago the clientele of most day centres and lunch clubs was relatively fit and independent—often able and willing to run the outfit themselves. While there is still a need to provide some form of service for this group, it is the very old, frail and often confused elderly who have a special need for day care. These are the people who may be housebound and who may rely heavily on one or two carers. Not only does day care encourage them to mix with other people and provide valuable social stimulation, but it allows the carers to have vital time to themselves.

It is our experience that the most successful day centres are small and local and are closely linked to the communities which they serve. While the role of volunteers is crucial to this success, we believe that in general such centres should have paid coordinators, particularly when many of the members are physically frail and confused. Paid staff and volunteers should have adequate training and support if they are to cater for this group. The needs of different communities vary enormously: the day centre which is ideal for a small village may not suit the rundown centre of a city or the suburb of a town.

The general practitioner can provide valuable support to a local day centre. He can also initiate discussions about a new project, if such a need has been identified. The lack of adequate day care in the community bedevils many geriatric and psychogeriatric day hospitals, which cannot discharge some patients who no longer require that form of care yet need day care of the sort provided in day centres and whose relatives certainly require 'time off'. This affects the efficiency of the hospital service and may lead to the unwelcome development of waiting lists for day-hospital attendance.

HOUSING

General practitioners may be asked to give advice on housing matters and to mediate on their patients' behalf with housing departments and housing associations. Often old people, their relatives and members of the primary care team believe that a change of house will solve all their current problems, and are surprised when this turns out to be untrue. It is important to identify the reasons why a person or a couple wish to move house. On the whole, it is preferable to avoid such a move if other solutions can be found, particularly if the move takes the old person far away from the community in which he/she has lived for most of his/her life. This is especially pertinent to those elderly people who uproot themselves to live in the seaside resort of which they harbour idyllic (and distorted?) holiday memories; or for elderly parents who move into 'granny flats' without due consideration for their previous relationship with the younger generation concerned.

The general practitioner should be prepared to act as 'devil's advocate'—putting forward the disadvantages of moving if he feels that his patient has not considered them fully. Important decisions of this sort should never be taken hurriedly and especially not in the aftermath of a crisis such as widowhood, when judgements of all concerned are apt to be adversely affected.

Many people regard 'housing for the elderly' as synonymous with 'sheltered housing'. In fact, the vast majority of old people live in ordinary houses, either owner-occupied or rented from the local authority, a housing association or a private landlord. Studies have shown that old people are more likely to live in 'sub-standard' housing, i.e. lacking such basic amenities as hot water, bath or shower, or inside toilet, than the general population.

Perhaps this is part of the reason that many people—old and young—believe that there should be considerably more sheltered housing, but even if the target figures for this special provision were achieved, only about 5 per cent of people aged over 65 would be housed in this way. In subsequent paragraphs we outline the advantages of sheltered housing, which certainly provides a package of support, in terms of bricks and mortar, combined with a personal service, which suits some old people very well. However, many others either do not need this package or do not want to move house at all. For them it may be more appropriate to consider home improvement grants, or the provision of more simple aids and adaptations (the advice of the domiciliary occupational therapy service is invaluable here), or perhaps the installation of an alarm call system.

Sheltered Housing

Sheltered housing schemes are grouped dwellings for the elderly which are specially designed for their needs. Usually there is a resident caretaker or warden with some form of communication system between each resident and the warden. The houses are centrally heated, and if built on more than one storey, a lift is usually provided. Some schemes offer extra facilities such as common sitting room/TV room, communal laundry, and rarely a communal dining room. Most of the apartments are designed for single tenants in which case they comprise living room, bedroom, kitchenette and bathroom. In some schemes there is a living room with a screened bed annexe described as 'one and a half rooms'. A few apartments are suitable for two persons, usually husband and wife, but occasionally sisters or lifelong friends.

Until recently, sheltered housing schemes were built and managed by local authority housing departments or housing associations and the houses were only available to rent. Over the past few years, the private sheltered housing market has flourished. It is important that elderly people who decide to buy an apartment in a private sheltered housing scheme should understand the contract which they undertake and the support to which they are entitled.

On the whole, the managers of sheltered housing schemes prefer to accept tenants or owner-occupiers who are reasonably independent. They also accept a certain degree of physical and mental deterioration thereafter, but it is important to remember that the warden's task is not to provide direct help for tenants but simply to fulfil a watching brief. She will put a daily call through to each tenant, to see that they are up and about; should problems arise, she knows when and how to summon appropriate help. Wardens will usually devise means of 'checking up' on tenants without obtrusiveness or conveying the impression that they are spying on their charges. Wardens are *not* expected to attend to tenants when they are afflicted by temporary illness or incapacity, although many will do so in a kind and neighbourly fashion. The help summoned by the warden will depend upon individual circumstances. Thus, where there is a concerned daughter nearby, she would be the obvious person to contact, while in other circumstances the warden would initially contact the general practitioner, the district nurse or home help supervisor as circumstances dictate.

It is very important that general practitioners and other primary carers fully appreciate the wardens' role and do not expect (and lead others to expect) high levels of direct help from them. This can readily happen as in the case of the warden who approached one of us to ask for advice. It transpired that one of her tenants had suffered a stroke and was nearly totally dependent. He was being looked after with great difficulty by his frail and elderly wife. After the general practitioner had visited the couple, the warden approached him in the expectation that the patient would be admitted to hospital. Instead she was told that it was her duty to nurse this old man and look after the apartment. This extreme case indicates the serious failure to understand that the warden is not a provider of direct support. As with other services, a friendly chat with the warden of a sheltered housing scheme will pay dividends for the general practitioner and the other primary team members.

Because the level of personal care available in sheltered housing is not significantly greater than that provided in ordinary housing, some old people need to move yet again into residential care or into long-term hospital care. Some of the organizations responsible for sheltered housing—particularly some of the housing associations—consider it unfortunate that an old frail person should be subjected to the anxiety and trauma of further moves. This has led to the development of 'extra care' sheltered housing, where quite heavily dependent residents may be suitably cared for by the provision of additional staff. These arrangements seem to work well and may provide an attractive alternative to residential care at present provided by local authorities. It may be argued that, by providing a wide range of support for tenants in sheltered housing, the family contribution may be diminished; this would have adverse effects since all studies have shown that the happiness and well-being of old people are closely related to the extent of family support. This has not yet been substantiated and, indeed, it may be that families are more prepared to help their elders when they share the support with other people.

We believe that the main benefit for tenants of sheltered housing is not to be found in its tangible elements such as special design and central heating. Rather it may be the more subtle advantage of the sense of security which tenants enjoy. An old person, on entering sheltered housing, is immediately aware that from there onwards if difficulties arise these will be identified and, it is to be hoped, something will be done. This is a powerful solace to old people since many, especially those living alone, harbour fears that 'something may happen'. Usually this 'something' is not specific but if pressed to explain this fear, they will ask: 'What happens if I become ill or cannot cope?' We believe that this is generally a sense of insecurity associated with a realization of increasing vulnerability and uncertainty of what to do and that no one would notice that things were going badly. Tenants in sheltered housing have the comforting feeling that, should they become ill or have a serious fall, it could never be more than a few hours before their predicament was recognized and help forthcoming.

VOLUNTARY ORGANIZATIONS

The statutory services—health and local authorities—are so called because they have obligations to provide specific services laid down in statute. Many try to widen their remits to provide more comprehensive services to vulnerable clients and their carers. Organizational difficulties and financial constraints often impede progress towards this goal.

Voluntary organizations usually develop in response to a perceived need which is not being met by the statutory sector. Because a voluntary body is not hidebound by bureaucracy, it should be able to behave in a flexible way to meet that need. Often the stimulus for its creation comes from 'the grass-roots', 'the consumers', rather than from 'the professionals'—particularly those who plan services at some distance from the point of delivery. However, there is a danger that voluntary initiatives may unwittingly overlap and still leave gaps in the provision of a comprehensive service. Ideally, voluntary organizations in a local area should take part in the planning process alongside the statutory bodies. This has the added advantage of injecting some 'grass-roots' opinion into a process which may otherwise easily become remote and centralized.

Some of the voluntary organizations are national, such as Age Concern, Help the Aged, British Association for Service to the Elderly, or local, such as the different crossroads schemes which have developed in many areas to provide sitting-in services for the carers of dependent relatives. Self-help groups have also been established to provide information and counselling services. The Alzheimer's Disease Society and the Parkinson's Disease Society are examples of this and the Chest, Heart and Stroke Association run local stroke clubs for patients with dysphasia. These groups may become very involved in campaigning, both locally and nationally. Voluntary organizations, representing the consumer as they do, are in a good position to lobby those who can bring about change.

Local communities, perhaps by way of church groups or residents' associations, can develop services on a small scale such as day centres, counselling and visiting services, good neighbour schemes and hospital transport services (although those voluntary schemes which have involved the use of private cars have become much less available as transport costs have increased). Such initiatives deserve support, and their organizers usually welcome encouragement from local general practitioners (who may themselves be the initiators of projects as they are in such a good position to identify the inadequacies of local services for their patients).

There is an enormous number of different voluntary organizations concerned with elderly people. Some may also work with other age groups. There are useful local and national directories which give information about them; the Citizens' Advice Bureau or the local Age Concern organizations are also useful sources of information.

THE GERIATRIC SERVICE

Many primary team members may be unaware that the UK is the only country with a soundly established specialist geriatric service. Others such as Canada, New Zealand and Sweden are now in the process of developing geriatric medicine, while the United States presently has a policy *not* to encourage what they have called a 'practice specialty' of geriatric medicine.

The history of British geriatric medicine is interesting since it stemmed to a large degree from the pioneering efforts of Dr Marjory Warren in the period 1935 to 1945. She showed that in old age accurate diagnosis and appropriate therapy would often lead to satisfactory recovery. Equally important, she demonstrated that even in such traditionally unpromising conditions as stroke, well-planned rehabilitation by therapists and other enthusiastic team members could very often secure satisfactory recovery of function and lead to full or partial independence. These may not sound very remarkable achievements today, but 40 years ago they were positively revolutionary since they attacked and set aside many strongly held negative concepts about old age in general and disease and disability in particular.

Later workers showed the value of community services, day hospitals, prevention and health education in relation to old age.

In the past 10 years changes of emphasis have taken place within the specialty, and different service models have developed in different parts of the country. Lively debate has occurred within the specialty and this, we believe, is a healthy sign.

Briefly, there are three models currently on offer:

1. The age-related service in which all patients over a certain age are dealt with by the geriatric service when hospital referral is called for. The usual 'cut-off point' is 'over 75' which means, of course, that many patients who need geriatric care but are aged 65–75 will be denied it. Likewise, some old patients who do not really need the special skills of the geriatric team may receive geriatric care. These are patients who, although they fulfil the age requirements for geriatric referral, have single circumscribed disease which can be perfectly well managed by general physicians or appropriate subspecialists. Thus the 76-year-old man who sustains a myocardial infarction while playing golf could readily be managed in the same way as a 65-year-old or 55-year-old patient with a similar condition.

2. The so-called 'integrated service' in which the geriatrician operates as a full member of the acute medical team but maintains a special interest in 'geriatric' patients, however defined. In this type of service older patients are admitted directly to an acute medical unit and thereafter those that need it will be transferred to the geriatric ward (or rehabilitation ward as it may be called). Some argue that this is not in the best interests of these geriatric patients, and indeed this was one of Marjory Warren's lessons, viz. that some old people often fared badly in acute wards, where equipment and furniture are often unsuitable and, most importantly, where nursing and other staff are not specially interested or trained in their special needs. The fact that some of them have to be moved to another ward to complete their treatment and rehabilitation can often have a delaying and sometimes prejudicial effect, since they have to

adjust to a new environment, get to know new staff and learn all over again how to 'operate the system'.

3. The 'selected referral' model in which patients are referred because they need the skills of the geriatric team. This decision is left to the general practitioner who thus fulfils his customary 'gate-keeping' role.

For our part, we favour the selected referral system of geriatric provision because we believe that where well organized it offers the best chance of ensuring that patients with geriatric needs receive geriatric care. Working in this way we find our work interesting, challenging and totally absorbing. We feel that it leaves us little time or energy to be dabbling in other branches of medicine.

Whatever model is chosen, it is essential that the services should be highly community orientated since 98 per cent of old people are not in hospital at any given time. This means close collaboration with general practitioners and other primary carers. It is the responsibility of the geriatrician to inform practitioners of the workings of their service. Personal contact between staff members in the geriatric service and primary care workers should be encouraged, so that the consultants, ward and day-hospital nursing staff become much more than names on letters or voices on the telephone. Most geriatric units have competent secretaries who are often the first contact for general practitioners or others seeking help for patients; these secretaries are worth getting to know also.

General practitioners may sometimes be unsure whether an individual patient should be first referred to the geriatric service, psychogeriatric service or social services. Such uncertainty is not surprising since the precise identification of need may be difficult—that is one reason why specialism has occurred. We tell our general practitioner colleagues that if there are doubts then the patient should be referred to the geriatric service.

A good geriatric service should offer the following items:

1. Home visits, sometimes in the company of the general practitioner (theoretically ideal but often difficult to arrange and can lead to delays in bringing help as mutually convenient times may be difficult to find)
2. Outpatient attendance
3. Day-hospital attendance
4. Inpatient care

The advantages of home visits and seeing patients in their own environments have already been stressed in several preceding sections.

Outpatient attendance requires little extra mention but it is worth discussing more fully day-hospital and inpatient services.

The Geriatric Day Hospital

This offers the opportunity to carry out full medical investigation, multidisciplinary team assessment and rehabilitation while avoiding admission to the wards. The day hospital also often facilitates earlier discharge for patients who have had to be admitted.

This is another service which has greatly expanded in recent decades—from only a handful in the early sixties to over 300 in 1980.

While we regard our day hospital as a most valuable resource, it is also extremely expensive, each patient visit costing in the region of £25–30 (at 1985 prices). These costs have gone up steeply, partly due to the rapid increase in transport costs which now represent about 20 per cent of all day-hospital running expenses. Because of this high cost, it is essential that the day hospital should be used only for patients who genuinely need medical, nursing, therapeutic or rehabilitation services. Each patient should be reviewed regularly and the staff should pose themselves the question: 'What are we doing for this patient?' If the answer does not include one or more of the above items, then the patient should be discharged. Home patients should never attend solely for social reasons such as relief of loneliness for which other more appropriate help should be sought, such as voluntary help or day centre or lunch club attendance. This may sound harsh, but it is much harsher if an expensive day hospital is allowed to function as a cosy social club for an elderly local élite and thereby its resources denied to other needy patients who could benefit enormously from its help.

Geriatric Inpatient Care

This may be required for diagnosis and treatment as in any other clinical service, but it also invariably involves multidisciplinary assessment and the provision of a suitable programme of rehabilitation for each patient. In order to achieve these aims, the geriatric service should have ready access to a full range of diagnostic and therapeutic facilities, which means that it should be based upon a general hospital. While there is some debate about the benefits of 'high technology' medicine for older patients, there can be no doubt about the advantages to them of such measures as joint replacement, cardiac pacemakers and modern endoscopic techniques. It could be argued that a teaching hospital, which, near the end of the twentieth century, does not have an active geriatric unit within it, is unlikely to be meeting the educational needs of medical and other students who will be practising in the next century.

A modern geriatric unit should also offer respite care both for simple 'holiday admission' purposes and as a recognition of the value of a firm offer to share the burden of care with hard-pressed relatives. We are very happy to offer regular, guaranteed admissions (2–3 weeks at a time usually) for families who wish to continue care at home but feel that they can face this more readily with this sort of relief. The old people concerned respond well to this service, especially if efforts are made to try to ensure that they return each time to the same environment and hence get to know nurses and therapists as 'old friends'. In over 25 years we have never been let down by relatives welching on the agreement and refusing to resume their care nor have we ever felt that patients had been harmed. Occasionally (1–2 per cent of cases) patients have died during a respite admission, but this is felt to be inevitable since most of them are very frail and death may intervene at any time. In such instances, considerable efforts are made to reassure relatives and assuage guilty feelings. Most old people are well aware that respite care makes it more feasible for their families to continue their supportive roles.

The geriatric service also provides continuing care for patients who cannot go home because of either severe dependency or inadequacy of home support (or a combination of these two factors). We prefer to provide this long-term care in wards set aside for this purpose and staffed by nurses and others who see their task as a special challenge and hence take special pride in making the lives of these patients as pleasant and non-institutional as possible. This is a difficult form of nursing care and it requires unusual attributes since the staff are usually denied the satisfaction of seeing patients get better and go home. The creation of a homely atmosphere, the arrangements for recreational and diversional activities require great imagination and ingenuity. In the earlier stages of a patient's stay in a continuing care ward, relatives may experience guilt and may react to this by being overcritical and demanding. We have often been impressed at the patience and resilience of ward staff in the face of what most would regard as selfish and unacceptable behaviour.

We discourage general practitioners and others from referring patients for long-term care for the very good reason that it is impossible to tell in advance of full assessment, treatment and rehabilitation which patients will end up in need of this type of care. If, however, a practitioner tells relatives that an old person should be in long-term care, then expectations are created which may not be fulfilled, e.g. where the patient makes a good (but unexpected) recovery as either a day patient or inpatient. It is much better (and more accurate) simply to tell patient and family that the help of the geriatrician is being sought.

Ideally, continuing care units should be small and local, situated within the community to which the patients belong, rather than centralized in large hospitals. Some units are staffed by local general practitioners and are visited regularly by geriatricians. This provides stability of medical cover (when compared with the often rapid turnover of junior doctors) and strengthens the existing links between the community and the unit, and between the general practitioners and the geriatrician.

Other Activities of the Geriatric Service

A good geriatric service will also be anxious to secure appropriate care for those 'geriatric' patients who need the skills of the geriatrician but who, for any reason, have found their way into other departments. This applies especially to general medicine, orthopaedic surgery and psychiatry. By importing the geriatric approach and team assessment for these patients, we have shown that they have a shorter stay in hospital and are more likely to go directly home (Burley *et al.* 1979). We recommend the establishment of geriatric/orthopaedic rehabilitation arrangements within the control of the geriatric service. Old patients, especially ladies with hip fractures, can be transferred thereto as soon after surgery as possible. In this way they have a better chance of early and successful rehabilitation, followed by day-hospital care where indicated.

PSYCHOGERIATRIC SERVICE

Some years after the benefits of a specialist geriatric service had been recognized, similar developments began to occur in psychiatry and there are now several hundred British psychiatrists who have geriatric psychiatry as their sole or principal interest.

This service has developed along similar lines to geriatric medicine. Generally patients fall into two main groups:

1. 'Organic' patients, i.e. those with dementia
2. 'Functional' patients, mostly with mood disorders

Psychogeriatric and geriatric services must work closely together and a variety of arrangements have been used to achieve this. Joint assessment units, regular combined ward rounds, shared outpatient or day-patient sessions have all shown value. Where the geriatric and psychogeriatric services share the same catchment areas and the respective consultants agree on mutual support, successful cooperation will usually follow. However, where one service is highly organized and well resourced, while the other has neither of these advantages, the more fortunate service will soon find itself doing some of the work of the less well endowed and resentment can ensue.

As with its geriatric counterpart, the psychogeriatric day hospital fulfils a diagnostic, assessment, therapeutic and rehabilitative role, especially for 'functional' patients in whom recovery is to be anticipated. For the 'organic' group, however, the day hospital's function is more custodial since recovery is rare or unusual in these patients.

In most areas, resources for dementia are seriously inadequate and become more so year by year due to the increasing numbers of aged persons. Since the prevalence of dementia is highly correlated with age and since the most aged groups are increasing most rapidly, it seems to us very probable that the 'rising tide' of dementia may engulf geriatric, general medical and social services in the next two decades unless very determined and substantial efforts are made. Another imponderable factor is the possibility that some pharmacological advance may occur which could improve function in sufferers from Alzheimer-type dementia. Even quite small improvements in cognitive function could enable an elderly patient to stay out of institutional care a little longer.

General practitioners, more than all others, must be aware of the great stresses generated by some demented patients among their families (and even among their neighbours). Not only their sons and daughters are affected but grandchildren may also be involved, and even after the patient is 'safely' in hospital or residential home (or, indeed, after death), tensions and feelings of guilt may persist.

Some psychiatrists have argued (from research experience) that there is little point in trying to keep demented old people at home if they have reached the stage of not being able to cope at home and have no relatives because such an attempt is bound to fail. Hence, if this argument is accepted, it is better to admit these patients as soon as possible and thereafter concentrate scarce community and day-care resources upon helping patients who do have caring relatives, since these are the only ones in whom success can be achieved. While this is probably mostly true, there are exceptions and we would argue that each case should be as fully assessed as possible and judged on individual merits.

SUMMARY AND CONCLUSION

This chapter has been provided because we believe that many doctors (and not, by any means, only general practitioners) and other primary team members have inadequate and often inaccurate knowledge of

PRIMARY CARE OF THE ELDERLY: A PRACTICAL APPROACH

important services, how to use them, for what kinds of patients and in what circumstances. We have therefore tried to outline some of these services and discuss how they have evolved and some of the inefficiencies and anachronisms which exist.

We hope that our effort will help primary care teams to find their way through the morass of local authority services, health services and voluntary services which exists.

We would like to conclude with a simple suggestion to the effect that practices might establish a 'glossary of services' for their own area. This would have several sections with subsections, more or less in the way we have indicated heretofore. Brief résumés of each service's responsibility would be succeeded by details of how to contact each one, e.g. telephone numbers, hours of access and names of key personnel. Perhaps some energetic practice manager has already done this—if so we would like to hear about it.

REFERENCES

Burley L. E., Currie C. T., Smith R. G. *et al.* (1979) Contribution from geriatric medicine within acute medical wards. *Br. Med. J.* **2**, 90.
Thompson M. K. (1984) *The Care of the Elderly in General Practice.* Edinburgh, London, Melbourne, New York: Churchill Livingstone.

GLOSSARY OF DRUGS

Glossary of drugs for the convenience of North American readers. Some terms which may be unfamiliar are fully explained in Chapter 9 (Services for the Elderly), e.g. district nurse, chiropodist etc.

Name used in text	UK proprietary name	N. American name (proprietary in brackets)
allopurinol	Zyloric	allopurinol (Zyloprin)
amantadine	Symmetrel	amantadine (Symonetrel)
amitriptyline	Tryptizol, Triptafen	amitriptyline (Eleval)
ampicillin	Penbritin, Amfipen	ampicillin (Ampicin, Penbritin)
atenolol	Tenormin	atenolol (Tenormin)
bendrofluazide	Neo-naclex	bendroflumethiazide (Naturetin)
benztropine	Cogentin	benztropine (Cogentin)
betahistine	Serc	betahistine (Serc)
bromocriptine	Parlodel	bromocriptine (Parlodel)
bumetanide	Bumex	bumetanide (Bumex)
captopril	Capoten	captopril (Capoten)

Name used in text	UK proprietary name	N. American name (proprietary in brackets)
chloral	Noctec	chloral (Noctec)
chlordiazepoxide	Librium	chlordiazepoxide (Librium)
chlormethiazole	Heminevrin	not available
chlorpromazine	Largactil	chlorpromazine (Largactil)
cimetidine	Tagamet	cimetidine (Tagamet)
cinnarizine	Stugeron	not available
clofibrate	Atromid-S	clofibrate (Atromid-S)
colchicine		colchicine
co-trimoxazole	Bactrim, Septrin	co-trimoxazole (Bactrim, Septra)
coumarin	Warfarin	dicouminarol (Warfarin)
diazepam	Valium	diazepam (Valium)
dichloralphenazone	Welldorm	dichloralphenazone (Chloralol)
digitoxin	Digitalina Nativelle	not available
emepronium bromide	Cetiprin	not available
ethacrynic acid	Edecrin	ethacrynic acid (Edicrin)
flucloxacillin	Fluclox	flucloxacillin (Fluclox)
flurazepam	Dalmane	flurazepam (Dalmane)
frusemide	Lasix	frusemide (Lasix)
gentamicin	Genticin	gentamicin (Garamycin)
imipramine	Tofranil	imipramine (Tofranil)
indomethacin	Indocid	indomethacin (Indocid)

Name used in text	UK proprietary name	N. American name (proprietary in brackets)
labetalol	Trandate	labetalol (Trandate)
lignocaine	Lidocaine	lignocaine (Lidocaine)
lorazepam	Ativan	lorazepam (Ativan)
lormetazepam	Noctamid	not available
madopar	Madopar	not available
metoclopramide	Maxolon	metoclopramide (Maxeran)
metoprolol	Betaloc	metoprolol (Betaloc)
mianserin	Bolvidon	mianserin (Bolvidon)
nifedipine	Adalat	nifedipine (Adalat)
nitrazepam	Mogadon	nitrazepam (Mogadon)
nortriptyline	Aventyl	nortriptyline (Aventyl)
paracetamol	Panadol	acetaminophen (Tylenol)
prednisolone	many names	prednisolone (many names)
prochlorperazine	Stemetil	prochlorperazine (Stemetil)
propantheline bromide	Pro-banthine	propantheline bromide (Pro-banthine)
propranolol	Inderal	propanolol (Inderal)
selegiline	Eldepryl	not available
sinemet	Sinemet	sinemet
slow K	Slow K	slow K
streptomycin	Streptomycin	streptomycin
sulphonylurea		sulphonylurea

Name used in text	UK proprietary name	N. American name (proprietary in brackets)
tamoxifen	Nolvadex	tamoxifen (Nolvadex)
temazepam	Euhypnos	temazepam (Restoril, Euhypnos)
theophylline	Nuelin, Theo-dur	theophylline (Theo-dur)
thioridazine	Melleril	thioridazine (Mellaril)
tolbutamide	Rastinon	tolbutamide (Orinase)
trazodone	Molipaxin	trazodone (Desyrel)
triazolam	Halcion	triazolam (Halcion)
tryptophan	Optimax	not available

Index

189